ABC of
Clinical Rea        ibrary

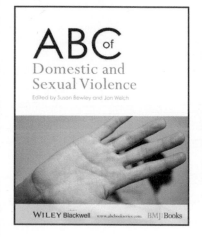
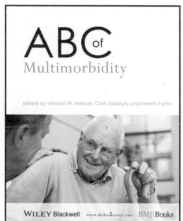
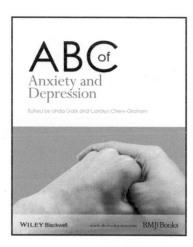
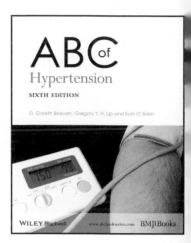
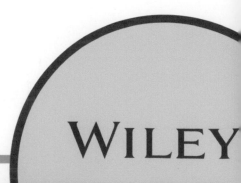

# ABC of

# Clinical Reasoning

EDITED BY

## Nicola Cooper

Consultant Physician and Honorary Clinical Associate Professor
Derby Teaching Hospitals NHS Foundation Trust and
Division of Medical Sciences and Graduate Entry Medicine,
University of Nottingham, UK

## John Frain

General Practitioner and Director of Clinical Skills
Division of Medical Sciences and Graduate Entry Medicine,
University of Nottingham, UK

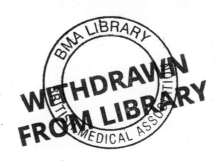

**WILEY** Blackwell          BMJ|Books

*Library of Congress Cataloging-in-Publication data applied for*

ISBN: 9781119059080

A catalogue record for this book is available from the British Library.

Wiley also publishes its books in a variety of electronic formats. Some content that appears in print may not be available in electronic books.

Cover image: © agsandrew/iStock

Set in 9.5/12pt Minion by SPi Global, Pondicherry, India

1    2017

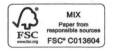

# Contents

# Contributors

**Maggie Bartlett**
MBChB FRCGP MA (medical education) SFHEA
Senior Lecturer in Medical Education, Keele School of Medicine, UK

**Nicola Cooper**
MBChB FAcadMEd FRCPE FRACP
Consultant Physician and Honorary Clinical Associate Professor,
Derby Teaching Hospitals NHS Foundation Trust and Division
of Medical Sciences and Graduate Entry Medicine, University
of Nottingham, UK

**Pat Croskerry**
MD PhD FRCPE
Director, Critical Thinking Program, Division of Medical Education,
Dalhousie University, Canada

**John Frain**
MBChB MSC FRCGP DCH DGM DRCOG PGDipCard
General Practitioner; Director of Clinical Skills, Division of
Medical Sciences and Graduate Entry Medicine, University of
Nottingham, UK

**Simon Gay**
MBBS FRCGP MSc MA (medical education) SFHEA
Senior Lecturer in Medical Education, Keele School
of Medicine, UK

**Martin Hughes**
MBChB BSc MRCP FRCA FFICM
Consultant in Anaesthesia and Intensive Care Medicine, Royal Infirmary,
Glasgow, UK

**Steven McGee**
MD
Professor of Medicine, University of Washington
General Medical Service
Department of Veterans Affairs Medical Center, Seattle, WA, USA

**Graham Nimmo**
MBChB BSc MD EdD FRCP(Edin) FFARCSI FFICM
Consultant in Intensive Care Medicine and Clinical Education
Western General Hospital, Edinburgh, UK

**Sian Powell**
MBChB MRCP MRCGP MA (Clin Ed)
GP and Course Lead for Year 6 General Practice Student Assistantship,
Department of Primary Care and Public Health, Imperial College School of
Medicine, Charing Cross Hospital, London, UK

**Ana L. Da Silva**
PhD AFHEA
Lecturer in Medical Education, Swansea University Medical School,
Swansea, UK

# Preface

Excellence in medicine is not just about good knowledge, skills and behaviours. How doctors think, reason and make decisions is arguably their most critical skill. While medical schools and postgraduate training programmes teach and assess the knowledge and skills required to practise as a doctor, few offer comprehensive training in clinical reasoning or decision-making. This is important because studies suggest that diagnostic error is common and results in significant harm to patients. Diagnostic error typically has multiple causes, but two-thirds of the root causes involve human cognitive error – most commonly, when the available data are not synthesised correctly. While some of this is due to inadequate knowledge, a significant amount is due to inadequate reasoning.

Clinical reasoning has several elements, which are covered in this book, from evidence-based clinical skills to the use and interpretation of diagnostic tests to cognitive psychology, thinking about thinking and human factors. This book is designed to be an introduction for individuals and also a resource for a curriculum in clinical reasoning.

Clinical reasoning is not confined to doctors – we have written this book with advanced nurse practitioners and other clinicians in mind, and try to use the word clinician' rather than 'doctor' whenever we can.

Clinical reasoning is relevant to every single specialty from general practice to surgery to the intensive care unit. While some aspects of clinical reasoning are not new, advances in cognitive psychology and a better understanding of patient safety mean there are elements of clinical reasoning that many clinicians may be unfamiliar with. We can only provide an introduction to the different elements of clinical reasoning in this book, so each chapter has a list of further reading and resources. We have also provided a list of recommended books, articles and websites at the end of the book so readers can continue to explore clinical reasoning in more depth for themselves.

We really enjoyed writing and editing this book, we hope you enjoy reading and using it!

**Nicola Cooper and John Frain**
**January 2016**

## CHAPTER 1

# Clinical Reasoning: An Overview

*Nicola Cooper[1,2] and John Frain[2]*

[1] Derby Teaching Hospitals NHS Foundation Trust, UK
[2] University of Nottingham, UK

---

**OVERVIEW**

- Clinical reasoning describes the thinking and decision-making processes associated with clinical practice

- The core elements of clinical reasoning include: evidence-based clinical skills, use and interpretation of diagnostic tests, understanding cognitive biases, human factors, metacognition (thinking about thinking), and patient-centred evidence-based medicine

- Diagnostic error is common and causes significant harm to patients. Errors in reasoning play a significant role in diagnostic error

- Sound clinical reasoning is directly linked to patient safety and quality of care

---

## Introduction

Fellow author, Pat Croskerry, argues that although there are several qualities we would look for in a good clinician, the two absolute basic requirements for someone who is going to give you the best chance of being correctly diagnosed and appropriately managed are these: someone who is both knowledgeable and a good decision-maker. At the time of writing, medical schools and postgraduate training programmes teach and assess the knowledge and skills required to practise as a doctor, but few offer a comprehensive curriculum in decision-making. This is a problem because how doctors think, reason and make decisions is arguably their most critical skill.

This book covers the core elements of clinical decision-making – or clinical reasoning. It is designed not only for individuals but also as an introductory text for a course or as part of a curriculum in clinical reasoning. Chapter 9 specifically covers teaching clinical reasoning in undergraduate and postgraduate settings. In this chapter we define clinical reasoning, explain why it is important, and provide an overview of the different elements involved.

## What is clinical reasoning?

Clinical reasoning describes the thinking and decision-making processes associated with clinical practice. According to Schön, it involves the 'naming and framing of problems' based on a personal understanding of the patient or client's situation. It is a clinician's ability to make decisions, often with others, based on the available clinical information, which includes history (sometimes from multiple sources), clinical examination findings and test results – against a backdrop of clinical uncertainty. Clinical reasoning also includes choosing appropriate treatments (or no treatment at all) and decision-making with patients and/or their carers. Box 1.1 gives a definition of clinical reasoning.

Figure 1.1 shows the different elements involved in clinical reasoning covered in this book, underpinned by a knowledge of basic and clinical sciences. Good clinical skills – in particular communication skills – are vital because the heart of the clinical reasoning process is often the patient's history and physical examination. Another element in clinical reasoning is understanding how to use and interpret diagnostic tests, something that is surprisingly rarely taught in a systematic way. Other elements include an understanding of cognitive psychology – how the human brain works with regards to decision-making – and human factors. We are unaware of the subconscious cognitive biases and errors to which we are prone in our everyday thinking and actions. Metacognition – thinking about thinking – is a critical skill that can be both learned and nurtured. It starts with an understanding of *how* we think, how our thinking and decision-making can be flawed, and how to mitigate this. Finally, reasoning does not end with a diagnosis. Patient-centred evidence-based medicine and shared decision-making (explored in Chapter 8) are also elements of clinical reasoning.

Clinical reasoning is a complex process that is not fully understood. It is only in recent years that doctors have begun to focus on their thinking processes, helped by advances in cognitive psychology that have given us models of decision-making that were

---

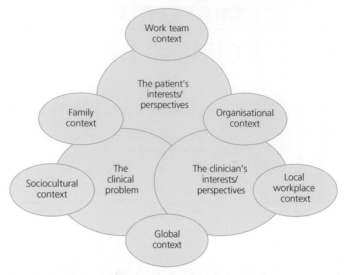

**Figure 1.2** Clinical reasoning in multiple problem spaces: factors influencing clinical decision-making. Source: Higgs J and Jones MA. Clinical decision making and multiple problem spaces. In: Higgs J, Jones MA, Loftus S, Christensen N (eds), *Clinical Reasoning in the Health Professions*, 3rd edn. Elsevier, 2008. Reproduced with permission of Elsevier.

**Table 1.1** Root causes of diagnostic error.

| Error category | Examples |
| --- | --- |
| No fault | Unusual presentation of a disease |
| | Missing information |
| System errors | Technical, e.g. unavailable tests/results |
| | Organisational, e.g. poor supervision of junior staff, error-prone processes, impossible workload |
| Human cognitive error | Faulty data gathering |
| | Inadequate reasoning |

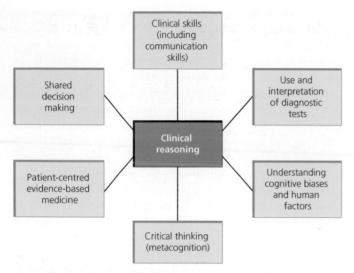

**Figure 1.1** The elements involved in clinical reasoning, underpinned by a knowledge of basic and clinical sciences.

not available before. In addition, while clinical reasoning is often conducted individually, it is often done in a team and also occurs in context – or 'problem spaces' as illustrated in Figure 1.2. These different contexts or *points of view* impact on our reasoning in ways we often do not realise.

## Why is clinical reasoning important?

Clinical reasoning is important because a wide variety of studies suggest that diagnostic error is common. Using various methods it is estimated that diagnosis is wrong 10–15% of the time, highest in the 'undifferentiated' specialties of emergency medicine, internal medicine and general practice. Diagnostic error causes significant harm – in the Harvard Medical Practice Study, which looked at adverse events, diagnostic error was much more likely to lead to serious disability than other types of error. In the USA, misdiagnosis now rivals surgical accidents as the leading cause of medico-legal claims.

There are many reasons why diagnostic error occurs. A comprehensive review of studies of misdiagnosis assigned three main categories, shown in Table 1.1. However, it has been estimated

that roughly two-thirds of the root causes of diagnostic error involve errors in reasoning, most commonly when the available data are not synthesised correctly. This means that sound clinical reasoning is directly linked to patient safety and quality of care, and teaching it should be a priority.

## History and examination

Clinical reasoning in medicine usually starts with a presenting complaint. We then listen to the patient's story – which could be from the patient or carers or eyewitnesses. During this process the clinician starts to generate different hypotheses as to what the problem might be. The history generates the most hypotheses. Clinical examination and in some cases tests narrow these down, as illustrated in Figure 1.3. For example, in breathlessness there is a wide differential. Experienced clinicians generate hypotheses early and are able to ask specific questions during the history in order to explore these hypotheses further. During the clinical examination the list of differentials becomes smaller if some findings are present or absent, and test results narrow things down even more – although as Chapter 3 explains, not in the way we might think.

Although students are taught history and examination skills there may be little emphasis on the evidence-base or context of

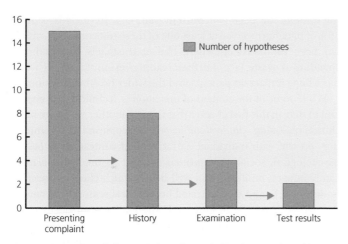

**Figure 1.3** Number of diagnostic hypotheses during the steps in making a diagnosis. Source: Sox HC, Higgins MC, Owens DK. *Medical Decision Making*. Wiley-Blackwell, Oxford, 2013. Reproduced with permission of John Wiley & Sons, Ltd.

these vital skills. We make many assumptions about history and examination – a topic that is explored further in Chapter 2.

## Probability and diagnostic tests

Information gathering can happen in seconds, as in the resuscitation room of an emergency department, or over a longer period of time, as in a clinic setting. After gathering information the clinician has to decide whether to treat, gather more information, or wait and see. Lots of factors come into play at this point: probability/odds, risks versus benefits, what is available, patient wishes and so on. Probability/odds (or to put it another way 'uncertainty quantified') is a key element in clinical reasoning and is present from start (history) to finish (discussing the pros and cons of a particular treatment). A definition of probability and odds is shown in Box 1.2.

Sox and colleagues (see 'Further reading/resources') state that the most fundamental principle in clinical decision-making is that *the interpretation of new information depends on what you believed beforehand*. In other words, the interpretation of a test result depends on the clinical probability of the disease before the test is performed. They go as far to say, 'Once you accept this principle, your life will never be the same again.' This principle again reinforces the importance of clinical skills – being able to elicit the patient's story and physical examination findings.

Tests are commonly misused by clinicians. We do not understand probabilities or the information we receive from tests. Tests change the probability of a particular disease being present or absent, but rarely in a binary yes/no fashion. More commonly a test will increase or decrease the likelihood of a disease being present by less than we think.

For example, CT angiography to diagnose ischaemic bowel is a good test – it is 94% specific and 93% sensitive. This combination of high sensitivity and high specificity is rare. But even with such a good test, if we are highly suspicious of ischaemic bowel (say a pre-test probability of 80%) then a negative test reduces the chance of ischaemic bowel to 20%. This is far from zero.

Spirometry testing in the community for chronic obstructive pulmonary disease (COPD) is common. The sensitivity of this test is 92% and the specificity 84%. If we believe a heavy smoker with persistent wheeze has COPD (say we think the pre-test probability is 90%) then a negative test still leaves a 46% chance the patient has COPD. If we are not sure about the diagnosis (say a 50% pre-test probability) a positive test changes the probability to 85% and a negative test to 9%.

In other words, the interpretation of new information depends on what you believed beforehand. The concepts of sensitivity, specificity, pre- and post-test probabilities, and so forth are explored in more detail in Chapter 3.

## Clinicians are human too

Even if we had the best knowledge and clinical skills our reasoning would still be flawed by virtue of the fact that we are human. Chapters 4, 5 and 6 explore this further. It is not a matter of intelligence or memory – the human brain is *wired* to miss things that are obvious, see patterns that do not exist, and jump to conclusions. We are also very poor at estimating probability. Clinicians are not exempt from these human characteristics. In his book *Human Error* (Cambridge University Press, 1990), psychologist James Reason argues that, 'Our propensity for certain types of error is the price we pay for the brain's remarkable ability to think and act intuitively – to sift quickly through the sensory information that constantly bombards us without wasting time trying to work through every situation anew.'

Humans have a fast, pattern recognising way of decision-making, and a slower more deliberate method of decision-making – often referred to as intuitive and analytical. Psychology and other disciplines have explored this 'two minds hypothesis', or dual process theory, which is explained further in Chapter 4.

Thinking itself is prone to error. This affects everyone. Also, error is not randomly distributed – we systematically err in the same direction, which makes our mistakes predictable, but only to a degree. Even highly intelligent people fall into the same cognitive traps or cognitive biases. Croskerry has termed these *cognitive dispositions to respond* in certain ways in particular situations. Cognitive biases are explored further in Chapter 5.

Human factors approaches this problem from a systems point of view. Research shows that errors are predictable and tend to repeat themselves in patterns. The systems in which we work, the processes that are in place, and how we communicate within teams can either adapt for this to make error less likely, or they can in fact create accidents waiting to happen. Unnecessarily complicated processes, fatigue and cognitive overload all impact on human performance. These 'affective biases' and the discipline of human factors is explained further in Chapter 6.

What can we do about our human tendency to err? Metacognition (thinking about thinking) and cognitive debiasing is explored in Chapter 7. Using guidelines, scores and decision aids – an area of increasing interest in an attempt to improve decision-making and patient safety – is explored in Chapter 8. Finally, the very important matter of how we can start to teach clinical reasoning in medical schools and in postgraduate training programmes is explored in Chapter 9.

## Clinical reasoning matters to patients

Diagnostic error definitely causes harm, but increasing attention is being paid to another problem in developed countries – the harm caused by unnecessary tests and *overdiagnosis*. Overdiagnosis occurs when people without relevant symptoms are diagnosed with a disease that ultimately will not cause them to experience symptoms or early death. There are many factors contributing to overdiagnosis (see Box 1.3), but one of the main ones is the increasing availability of increasingly sensitive tests.

A study of over one million Medicare patients looked at how often people received one of 26 tests or treatments deemed by scientific and professional organisations to be of no benefit (Shwarz A, Landon B, Elshaug A et al. Measuring low value care in Medicare. *JAMA Intern Med* 2014; 174:1067–76). These included things like brain imaging in syncope, screening for carotid artery disease in asymptomatic patients, and imaging of the spine in low back pain with no red flags. In one year at least 25% of patients received at least one of these tests or treatments. It has been estimated elsewhere that at least 20% of healthcare spending is waste (see 'Further reading/resources'). This waste has a huge impact on patients and the wider healthcare economy.

While some of the content of this book is 'technical' it is important to state in this first chapter that there is another vital element of clinical reasoning – *understanding people*. People are not machines, they present with individual narratives and context. They have a psychological, social and spiritual element to them that significantly impacts on illness and well-being, which clinicians need to understand. Figure 1.2 illustrated how clinical reasoning occurs in context. An example of context is the tendency of doctors and society to 'medicalise' people's problems. Research shows that labelling people with a diagnosis when in fact they are experiencing the normal trauma, anxiety and low mood that all humans experience can actually create illness. An example of this is given in Box 1.4. Medicine is often called an art as well as a science because it can be a very human and intuitive practice. Many studies demonstrate a correlation between effective clinician-patient communication (or 'whole person care') and improved health outcomes.

## Summary

It takes years to develop effective clinical reasoning skills. This is partly because clinical knowledge is a fundamental requirement for successful clinical reasoning and this takes years to acquire. However, as Chapter 9 ('Teaching Clinical Reasoning')

---

**Box 1.3 Factors contributing to overdiagnosis**

- Screening programmes that detect 'pseudodisease' – disease in a person without symptoms in a form that will never cause symptoms or early death
- Increasingly sensitive tests
- Greater access to scanning – diagnostic scanning of the head and body reveals incidental findings in up to 40% of those being scanned for other reasons, often leading to anxiety and further testing for an abnormality that would never have harmed them
- Widening definitions of disease and lower treatment thresholds, for example:
  - Chronic kidney disease
  - High cholesterol
  - Attention deficit hyperactivity disorder
- Cultural considerations - medicalisation, commission bias (better to do something than nothing), fear of litigation
- Individual clinicians' lack of understanding of statistics relevant to the disease, diagnostic test and intervention in question

Adapted from Moynihan R. Preventing overdiagnosis: how to stop harming the healthy. *BMJ* 2012; 344:e3502.

---

**Box 1.4 The tendency of doctors and society to 'medicalise' patients' problems**

Two patients had similar symptoms. They were experiencing transient numbness of different parts of the body – one side of the face or the other, sometimes the arm or hand. These symptoms were causing a great deal of anxiety. The patients went to see two different physicians who had different training, interests and perspectives (see Figure 1.2), so the outcome for the two patients was very different.

The first patient told his story. At the end of the consultation the physician said, 'Well you've either got migraine or multiple sclerosis so we'll do an MRI scan and I'll let you know the results.' He was not given a further appointment. While waiting for his MRI scan, his anxiety and symptoms increased significantly.

The second patient told her story. Recognising that these symptoms are common in stress and did not fit any neurological pattern, the physician said, 'I see lots of people with these symptoms and very often it's because they are working too hard, not sleeping, or under stress. Even though they might not realise they are stressed, their body is telling them they're stressed. Tell me about your schedule and what's going on in your life.' The patient's husband looked at her knowingly and sure enough there were lots of stressors related to work and home that had been an issue. An MRI scan was arranged, but the patient was advised to make changes to her lifestyle and her symptoms resolved.

Both patients had normal MRI scans.

Explanation and good communication leads to better outcomes, greater compliance with recommended treatment, and less re-attendances.

will explain, there are some other key ingredients that are required to develop expertise – for example coaching, deliberate practice and feedback. If we can start with an understanding of what clinical reasoning is, why it is important, what its key elements are and how to teach it, we can create clinicians who are better decision-makers and who ultimately provide better patient care.

## Further reading/resources

Berwick D and Hackbarth A. Eliminating waste in US healthcare. *JAMA* 2012; **307**(14):1513–6.

Graber ML. The incidence of diagnostic error in medicine. *BMJ Qual Saf* 2013; **22**:ii21–ii27.

Leape LL, Brennan TA, Laird NM et al. The nature of adverse events in hospitalized patients: results of the Harvard Medical Practice Study ll. *N Engl J Med* 1991; **324**:377–84.

Neale G, Hogan H, Sevdalis N. Misdiagnosis: analysis based on case record review with proposals aimed to improve diagnostic processes. *Clin Med* 2011; **11**(4):317–21.

Schön DA. *The Reflective Practitioner: How Professionals Think in Action*. New York: Basic Books, 1983.

Sox HC, Higgins MC, Owens DK. *Medical Decision Making*, 2nd edn. Oxford: Wiley-Blackwell, 2013.

## CHAPTER 2

# Evidence-Based History and Examination

*Steven McGee[1] and John Frain[2]*

[1] University of Washington; and Department of Veterans Affairs Medical Center, Seattle, USA
[2] University of Nottingham, UK

---

> **OVERVIEW**
>
> - An evidence-based approach to clinical skills allows clinicians to quickly identify symptoms and signs that are diagnostically most accurate
> - The history should identify key symptoms and also take into account the natural history of the disease and the patient's context
> - The best measure of diagnostic accuracy is the likelihood ratio, a parameter that is easy to understand and apply
> - By using an evidence-based approach and likelihood ratios, clinicians can become more efficient, confident and accurate when approaching diagnosis of their patients

## Introduction

Evidence-based history and examination is a specific method of processing clinical information, one that surveys all information from the clinical encounter, compares it to a recognised diagnostic standard and quickly identifies those variables with the greatest diagnostic accuracy.

Around 80% of diagnoses are made from the history. This percentage has remained remarkably constant despite technological advances in medicine. The purpose of the history is the generation of a differential diagnosis that is sufficiently broad to include the actual diagnosis but focused enough to be tested by an appropriate physical examination and sometimes investigations. As well as being patient-centred, the history is a rich source of clinical data (see Figure 2.1), which when carefully explored by listening and the use of open questions allows the clinician to observe Osler's maxim, 'Listen to your patient, he is telling you the diagnosis'.

Listening to the patient should produce in the mind of the clinician a reasoned differential diagnosis comprising a leading hypothesis and two to three other conditions, including 'must not miss' disorders, all justifiable by the data gathered. These differentials should be tested and modified by further questioning and an evidence-led physical examination. For example, in patients with a fever and a cough, clinicians typically examine for the traditional findings of pneumonia (see Figure 2.2). In clinical reasoning terms,

however, clinicians should wonder whether one finding is more accurate than another. Does each of these 15 findings increase the probability of pneumonia when present? Does each decrease the probability when absent? Do they all change the probability by an equal amount? Are some findings accurate and others not? This chapter aims to explore how we can think differently about history and examination from an evidence-based point of view.

## Evidence-based history

When gathering clinical information in a history, we can describe key symptoms within each system, as Box 2.1 illustrates. While symptoms may overlap different systems (e.g. chest pain could be cardiac or respiratory in origin) or be challenging for both patient and doctor to define (e.g. dizziness) many diseases within a body system present as variations of the key symptoms of that system. Provided the clinical setting of an individual symptom is clearly defined (e.g. nausea and vomiting in patients with suspected intestinal obstruction, or central chest pain in patients with suspected myocardial infarction) it is possible to calculate its statistical significance and thus its usefulness as evidence of the presence of the target condition.

Several studies have looked at features in the history that might be more diagnostic than others for a particular condition. One interesting study looked at what features of the history in *acute* chest pain are most helpful to clinicians in differentiating cardiac from non-cardiac causes (Swap CJ and Nagurney JT. Value and limitations of chest pain history in the evaluation of patients with suspected acute coronary syndromes. *JAMA* 2005; 294:2623–9). What the authors found was that no single element of the chest pain history was a powerful enough predictor of non-cardiac pain to allow a clinician to make a decision on history alone. But researchers have attempted to combine features in the history that can be of use in clinical practice – see Box 2.2. Pain that is stabbing, pleuritic, positional or reproducible by palpation has likelihood ratios near zero, meaning the likelihood of this kind of pain being cardiac is very low. Conversely, chest pain that radiates to one or both shoulders or arms or is precipitated by exertion has higher likelihood ratios (2.3–4.7), meaning this kind of pain is

---

*ABC of Clinical Reasoning*, First Edition. Edited by Nicola Cooper and John Frain.

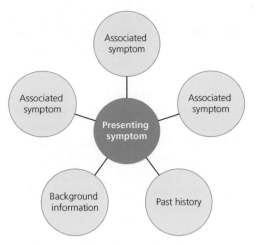

**Figure 2.1** Configuration of the symptoms of a patient's presentation.

| Traditional findings | Evidence-based approach |
|---|---|

**Traditional findings**

Fever
Tachypnoea
Tachycardia
Reduced oxygen saturation
Grunting respirations
Cyanosis
Asymmetric chest excursion
Percussion dullness
Diminished breath sounds
Crackles
Aegophony
Bronchophony
Whispering pectoriloquy
Bronchial breath sounds
Pleural rub

**Evidence-based approach**

5 findings *increase* probability

Asymmetrical chest excursion
Aegophony
Bronchial breath sounds
Percussion dullness
Oxygen saturation <95%

1 finding *decreases* probability

All vital signs normal

**Figure 2.2** Diagnosis of lobar pneumonia. Textbooks present 15 traditional physical findings of pneumonia (*left*), along with the assumption that each finding has similar diagnostic weight. The evidence-based method (*right*), based on study of actual patients, shows that five findings accurately increase probability of pneumonia, and only one finding decreases it.

---

**Box 2.1 Summary of key symptoms by body system**

**General**
- Fatigue/malaise
- Fevers/rigors/night sweats
- Weight/appetite
- Sleep disturbance
- Rashes/bruising

**Cardiovascular**
- Pain
- Breathlessness
- Palpitations
- Swelling

**Respiratory**
- Pain
- Breathlessness
- Wheeze
- Cough
- Sputum/haemoptysis

**Alimentary**
- Difficulty swallowing
- Nausea/vomiting/haematemesis
- Indigestion/heartburn
- Pain/distension
- Change in bowel habit
- Bleeding

**Genitourinary**
- Frequency
- Dysuria
- Incontinence
- Change in urinary volume
- Prostatic symptoms
- Menstrual symptoms

**Nervous system**
- Headache
- Loss of consciousness
- Dizziness
- Visual disturbance
- Hearing
- Weakness
- Numbness/tingling
- Memory or personality change
- Anxiety/depression

**Musculoskeletal**
- Pain
- Stiffness
- Swelling
- Loss of function or activities of daily living

Adapted from the Calgary-Cambridge Guide to the Medical Interview. In: Van Dalen J, Silverman J, Kurtz S, Draper J. *Skills for Communicating with Patients*, 3rd edn. Abingdon: Radcliffe Publishing, 2013.

---

more likely to be cardiac. Likelihood ratios (defined in Figure 2.3) are a useful tool in evidence-based history and examination and are explained in more detail later.

## Natural history and context

'Classical' presentations of disease are actually quite uncommon. The *natural history* of a disease is the sequence of changes that occur within the body and the patient's experience of it from the beginning of the illness to the end. Some symptoms and signs occur early in the disease while others occur later. For example, in the early stages of heart failure, the patient may only become short of breath on severe exertion. Later, breathlessness occurs on more moderate exertion (e.g. climbing the stairs), while later still the patient has a problem lying flat in bed and may be breathless even at rest.

If a junior clinician interviewing a patient with breathlessness believes the symptoms of orthopnoea must be present for the diagnosis of heart failure to be made, he or she is going to miss patients in the earlier stages of the disease who may benefit from proven treatment. This combination of the patient's presenting

$$\text{Likelihood ratio} = \frac{\text{Probability of finding in patients } with \text{ disease}}{\text{Probability of finding in patients } without \text{ disease}}$$

Examples:

(1) *Detecting pneumonia:* In patients with acute respiratory complaints, "percussion dullness" is found in 18% of patients with pneumonia and in 6% patients with another cause of respiratory distress. Therefore,

$$LR \left( \begin{array}{l} \text{for percussion dullness} \\ \text{in detecting pneumonia} \end{array} \right) = \frac{18}{6} = 3.0$$

(2) *Detecting coronary artery disease:* In patients with chronic chest pain, "dysphagia" is reported in 4% of patients found to have coronary disease and in 20% of patients with another cause of chest pain. Therefore,

$$LR \left( \begin{array}{l} \text{for dysphagia} \\ \text{in detecting coronary} \\ \text{artery disease} \end{array} \right) = \frac{4}{20} = 0.2$$

**Figure 2.3** Likelihood ratios: definition and examples. McGee's Evidence Based Physical Diagnosis, 3rd Edition 2012.

symptoms and the natural history of the condition is reflected in the New York Heart Association's Functional Classification of Heart Failure (see Table 2.1). The approximate correlates of each class with echocardiographic findings can be used to guide evidence-based therapy.

The patient's context, including age and gender, should be emphasised when considering pre-test probabilities of a disease. Epidemiological studies help to provide the history with an evidence base to assist clinical reasoning. For example, as the INTERHEART study illustrated (see 'Further reading/resources'), cardiac chest pain is more likely in an older person who smokes, with a history of diabetes and high cholesterol, than in a young woman with no cardiac risk factors.

## Evidence-based physical examination

In the previous example of physical examination of patients with possible pneumonia, an evidence-based approach answers the question, 'What findings most accurately increase the probability of pneumonia?' by studying patients with respiratory complaints and comparing their physical examinations to chest radiographs. Based on evaluation of over 6000 patients, this approach concluded that six traditional physical findings reliably predict the results of the chest radiograph (as illustrated in Figure 2.2). The remaining findings, whether present or absent, add very little to the diagnosis of pneumonia. Using an evidence-based approach can trim the clinician's focus from 15 findings of unknown value to six findings with proven value, thereby increasing confidence, efficiency and accuracy. Clinicians applying this method can then approach their next patient with cough and dyspnoea as if they had personally examined each of the 6000 patients in these studies and then recalled the value of the physical examination gleaned from that experience.

## Using likelihood ratios

To use evidence-based methods, clinicians require a measure of diagnostic accuracy that is simple to understand and apply. Such a measure is the likelihood ratio (LR). Each finding from the history, examination or a test result is associated with a unique LR, a number whose values range from 0 to infinity. An LR greater than 1.0 *increases* the probability of disease, and the greater the value of the LR, the greater the increment in probability. Likelihood ratios are therefore 'diagnostic weights' – see

**Table 2.1** New York Heart Association Functional Classification of Heart Failure – assessment of the patient's functional status in the history is crucial in guiding therapy and correlates with prognosis.

| Class | I | II | III | IV |
|---|---|---|---|---|
| **Symptoms** | None | Slight limitation of physical activity | Marked limitation of physical activity | At rest and unable to perform activity without symptoms |
| **Maximum ejection fraction** | <45% | <45% | <35–45% | <35–45% |
| **Consider these drugs with appropriate monitoring** | ACE inhibitor or angiotensin-receptor blocker (ARB) Beta-blocker | ACE inhibitor or ARB Beta-blocker Loop diuretic | ACE inhibitor or ARB Beta-blocker Loop diuretic Aldosterone antagonist | ACE inhibitor or ARB Aldosterone antagonist Loop diuretic Beta-blocker (if compensated) |

Adapted from 2013 ACCF/AHA Guideline for the Management of Heart Failure: A Report of the American College of Cardiology Foundation/American Heart Association Task Force on Practice Guidelines. *Circulation* 2013; **128**:e240–e327.

Figure 2.4. An LR of less than 1.0 *decreases* the probability of disease. The closer the value of LR is to zero, the greater the reduction in probability. LRs whose values are close to 1.0 describe unhelpful findings because they do not change the probability at all.

One simple method of interpreting LRs is to memorise the association between three LR values – 2, 5 and 10 – and the first three multiples of 15 – 15, 30 and 45. A finding with an LR of 2 increases the absolute probability by around 15% (i.e. the clinician *adds* 15% to the pre-test probability); a finding with an LR of 5 increases the probability by around 30%, and one with an LR of 10 increases the probability by around 45%. This is illustrated in Table 2.2.

For those LRs less than 1.0, the clinician simply inverts the 2, 5, and 10 'rule' (i.e. 0.5, 0.2 and 0.1). A finding with an LR of 0.5 decreases the probability by around 15%; one with an LR of 0.2 decreases the probability by around 30%, and one with an LR of 0.1 decreases the probability by around 45%. As long as clinicians round off final probabilities greater than 100% to 100%, and those less than 0% to 0%, this method suffices for the purposes of clinical reasoning.

Table 2.2 summarises the absolute changes in probability for the most commonly used LRs. Findings with LRs greater than 3 or less than 0.3 are most helpful because these values identify findings that either increase or decrease probability by 20–25% or more.

## The limitations of evidence-based history and examination

There are two caveats to recognise before applying evidence-based history and examination to clinical reasoning. First, this method is appropriate only when the clinical problem is defined by a technological diagnostic standard, such as laboratory testing or clinical imaging (see Figure 2.5). Examples of such disorders, and their technological standards, are pneumonia (compared with chest radiographs), ascites (ultrasonography), coronary artery disease (coronary angiography), anaemia (full blood count), and hyperthyroidism (thyroid function tests). In each of these disorders, the evidence-based approach compares findings from the history or examination to the accepted technological standard and identifies the findings that most accurately predict the results of that standard. However, because many clinical problems lack technological standards, evidence-based reasoning is not always applicable. For these problems, empirical observation – what the clinician sees, feels and hears at the bedside – remains the sole diagnostic standard and LRs cannot be calculated.

**Table 2.2** Likelihood ratios and bedside estimates.

| Likelihood ratio | Approximate change in probability[a] |
| --- | --- |
| 0.1 | −45% |
| 0.2 | −30% |
| 0.3 | −25% |
| 0.5 | −15% |
| 1 | No change |
| 2 | +15% |
| 3 | +20% |
| 4 | +25% |
| 5 | +30% |
| 6 | +35% |
| 7 | |
| 8 | +40% |
| 9 | |
| 10 | +45% |

[a]These changes describe *absolute* increases or decreases in probability (from McGee S. Simplifying likelihood ratios. *J Gen Intern Med* 2002; **17**:646–9).

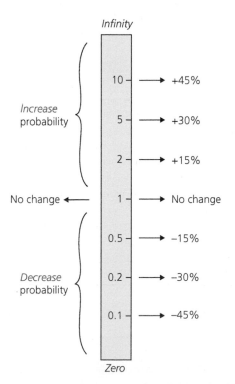

**Figure 2.4** Likelihood ratios: diagnostic weights. Clinicians should classify LRs into three groups: those with values greater than 1.0 increase probability; those with values less than 1.0 decrease probability; and those with values near 1.0 change probability very little or not at all.

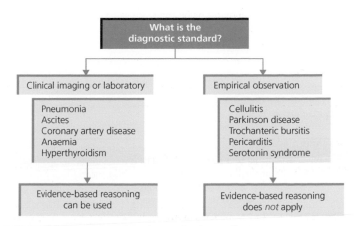

**Figure 2.5** Can evidence-based reasoning be used?

A second caveat is that evidence-based history and examination is not 'cookbook medicine'. Even though it describes how probability changes, *it cannot determine the pre-test probability of a disease*. For example, the LR for the physical finding 'fluid wave' in detecting ascites in patients with abdominal distension is 5.0 (a +30% probability). If the clinician works in a hepatology practice in which 60% of all patients with abdominal distension have ascites (i.e. a pre-test probability of 60%) the finding of a fluid wave is diagnostic (i.e. 60% + 30%, or a 90% probability of ascites). On the other hand, if the clinician works in a community practice where only 20% of patients with abdominal distension have ascites (the other 80% have increased abdominal fat or gas), the presence of the fluid wave is less conclusive (20% + 30%, or a 50% probability of ascites). Despite its name, evidence-based history and examination is much more than rote computation, because its proper application requires intimate knowledge of the types of disorders usually found in one's own practice.

## Example: diagnosing stable coronary artery disease

LRs allow clinicians to quickly compare many findings simultaneously, pinpointing those that have the greatest accuracy. For example, Table 2.3 reviews an evidence-based approach to the diagnosis of stable coronary artery disease in outpatients with chronic, intermittent chest pain (the diagnostic standard is coronary angiography). The first column of Table 2.3 identifies the clinical variable, the second column the number of patients studied, and the final columns provide the LRs for when the finding is present or absent. The LR when a finding is present is often labelled a 'positive LR'; the LR when finding is absent is often labelled a 'negative LR'. Statistical analyses and confidence intervals (which provide information about the strength of evidence) are omitted to simplify the presentation.

To quickly identify those findings that increase the probability of coronary artery disease the most, the clinician simply looks for

**Table 2.3** Diagnosing coronary artery disease in patients with stable, intermittent chest pain.

| | No. of patients | LR if the finding is: Present | Absent |
|---|---|---|---|
| Classification of chest pain:[a] | | | |
| Typical angina | 11,544 | 5.8 | – |
| Atypical angina | 11,182 | 1.2 | – |
| Non-anginal chest pain | 11,182 | 0.1 | – |
| Other pain characteristics: | | | |
| Burning pain | 250 | NS | NS |
| Better with glyceryl trinitrate within 5 minutes | 626 | 1.8 | 0.7 |
| Associated dyspnoea | 250 | NS | NS |
| Associated dysphagia | 130 | 0.2 | NS |
| Duration of pain <5 minutes | 130 | 2.4 | 0.2 |
| Duration of pain >30 minutes | 130 | 0.1 | NS |
| Risk factors: | | | |
| Male sex | 17,593 | 1.6 | 0.3 |
| Age (years) | | | |
| <30 | 14,569 | NS | – |
| 30–49 | 15,681 | 0.6 | – |
| 50–70 | 15,481 | 1.3 | – |
| >70 | 15,266 | 2.6 | – |
| Hypertension | 1478 | NS | NS |
| Diabetes mellitus | 1478 | 2.3 | 0.9 |
| Current/past tobacco use | 1478 | 1.5 | 0.7 |
| Hyperlipidaemia | 1920 | 2.2 | 0.6 |
| Family history of coronary disease | 1003 | NS | NS |
| Prior myocardial infarction | 8216 | 3.8 | 0.6 |
| Physical examination: | | | |
| Earlobe crease | 1338 | 2.3 | 0.6 |
| Arcus senilis | 200 | 3.0 | 0.7 |
| Ankle-brachial index <0.9 | 1005 | 4.0 | 0.8 |
| Electrocardiogram normal: | | | |
| Normal | 309 | NS | NS |

[a]'Typical angina' here is substernal discomfort, precipitated by exertion and improved with rest, glyceryl trinitrate (or both) in less than 10 minutes. 'Non-anginal chest pain' is unrelated to activity, unrelieved by glyceryl trinitrate, and otherwise not suggestive of angina. 'Atypical angina' is substernal discomfort with atypical features: glyceryl trinitrate not always effective, inconsistent precipitating factors, relieved after 15–20 minutes of rest.
NS, not significant (i.e. a 95% confidence interval includes the value of 1.0).
Data from Chun AA, McGee SR. Bedside diagnosis of coronary artery disease: a systematic review. *Am J Med* 2004; **117**:334–43; and McGee SR. *Evidence-Based Physical Diagnosis*, 3rd edn. Philadelphia: Saunders, 2012.

the LRs with the greatest values. They are typical angina – defined in Table 2.3 – (LR 5.8, or a +35% in probability), an ankle-brachial index of less than 0.9 (LR 4.0, or a +25% in probability), history of prior myocardial infarction (LR 3.8, or a +25% probability), and arcus senilis (LR 3.0, or a +20% probability). To identify those findings that decrease probability the most, the clinician looks for LRs whose values are closest to 0. They are non-anginal chest pain, duration of pain more than 30 minutes (both have LR 0.1, or a – 45% probability) and associated dysphagia (LR 0.2, or a – 30% probability). Other findings – atypical angina, associated dyspnoea, 'burning' pain and hypertension-are diagnostically unhelpful (NS, or not significant, indicating the finding's LR is statistically no different from the value of 1.0). LRs near the value of 1.0 imply the finding is found just as often in patients with coronary disease as in those with alternative causes of chest pain.

This approach confirms what many experienced clinicians already know – the *history* contains the most important diagnostic information, risk factors are less accurate than the patient's description of chest pain, and laboratory testing (e.g. the 12-lead electrocardiogram, or ECG) adds little to diagnosis in patients with stable, intermittent chest pain (the LR for a normal ECG is not significant).

## Combining clinical findings

Only individual clinical findings appear in Table 2.3. Can individual findings be combined? This is permitted if the clinician believes the two findings are *independent* of each other (independence implies that the LR for the first finding is the same whether or not the second finding is present). For example, typical angina (an LR of 5.8) and hyperlipidaemia (an LR of 2.2) are likely to be independent because the accuracy of a history of typical angina is unlikely to be affected by the presence or absence of hyperlipidaemia. To combine findings, the clinician can simply multiply the two individual LRs (5.8 × 2.2), the resulting product (12.7, or a +50% probability) becomes the LR for combined 'typical angina and hyperlipidaemia'. Alternatively, the clinician could first apply typical angina (LR of 5.8, or a +35% probability), then hyperlipidaemia (LR of 2.2, or a +15% probability) to obtain the increment in probability for the combined findings (35% + 15%, or a +50% probability).

Clinicians should not combine the LRs of more than two individual findings unless clinical studies have proven that the findings are independent. Also, if there is any possibility that the individual findings are dependent on each other, their LRs should not be combined (e.g. typical angina and 'duration of pain <5 minutes' should not be combined, because pain lasting less than 10 minutes after rest or glyceryl trinitrate is a criterion for stable typical angina here).

## Conclusions

Increasingly, researchers are comparing clinical findings to diagnostic standards to reveal LRs for a wide variety of clinical disorders (see 'Further reading/resources'). These authors apply specific criteria to the selection of studies, criteria now adopted by most biomedical journals and collectively referred to as the STARD criteria (STAndards of the Reporting of Diagnostic accuracy studies). The most important of the STARD criteria are:

- Both the test (clinical symptom, sign or laboratory test) and diagnostic standard are clearly defined.
- All enrolled patients have symptoms suggestive of the particular diagnosis under study.
- Determination of the test result is blinded from determination of the diagnostic standard.
- The study presents enough information to allow calculation of LRs and their confidence intervals.

Clinicians applying this evidence-based approach can streamline their approach to patients, focusing on those findings with greatest diagnostic accuracy, an approach that will increase diagnostic efficiency and reduce costs. Nonetheless this does have limitations. The relevant literature is patchy, difficult to find, and for many clinical problems is non-existent. Furthermore, even when a problem has been studied, conclusions often rest on relatively few patients (e.g. in Table 2.3, the LR for dysphagia is based on study of just 130 patients). Whether diagnostic accuracy depends on clinical technique is largely unaddressed, although the few studies on this subject show diagnostic accuracy with students as observers is the same as with specialists, as long as the finding is well-defined. Finally, most literature on the subject focuses on individual findings, although it is well known that expert clinicians typically combine many findings simultaneously when diagnosing disease.

Describing diagnostic accuracy using LRs is easy to understand and apply, and clinicians using this approach can quickly hone their clinical skills. In future studies of evidence-based history and examination, investigators should explore clinical problems not yet studied, combinations of findings and their accuracy, and how clinical observations predict prognosis and response to treatment, not just diagnosis.

## Further reading/resources

Chun AA and McGee SR. Bedside diagnosis of coronary artery disease: A systematic review. *Am J Med* 2004; **117**:334–43.

McGee S. Simplifying likelihood ratios. *J Gen Intern Med* 2002; **17**:646–9.

McGee SR. *Evidence-based physical diagnosis*, 3rd edn. Philadelphia: Saunders, 2012.

Simel D and Renniee D. *The rational clinical examination: Evidence-based clinical diagnosis*, 1st edn. New York: McGraw-Hill Professional, 2008.

Yusuf S, Hawken S, Ounpuu S et al. Effect of potentially modifiable risk factors associated with myocardial infarction in 52 countries (the INTERHEART study): case-control study. *Lancet* 2004; **364**:937–52.

# CHAPTER 3

# Using and Interpreting Diagnostic Tests

*Nicola Cooper*

Derby Teaching Hospitals NHS Foundation Trust; and University of Nottingham, UK

---

## OVERVIEW

- There is no such thing as a perfect test

- Tests results are affected by a number of factors that the clinician has to take into account

- The probability that a patient has a disease depends on the clinical (pre-test) probability and the sensitivity and the specificity of the test

- The prevalence of the disease in the patient's population affects the predictive value of the test

- Thresholds provide a useful way of thinking about whether a test should be performed at all

---

## Introduction

Doctors and other clinicians have to make decisions without definitive information a lot of the time because there is no such thing as a perfect diagnostic test. One of the characteristics of a medical professional is 'judgement in the face of uncertainty' (Royal College of Physicians of London, 2005). Even with a good test that has 90% sensitivity and 90% specificity, 10% of patients with the disease will have a normal test result and 10% of patients without the disease will have an abnormal test result. Tests have to be interpreted in the light of the patient's history and examination and are affected by a number of factors:
- Normal values
- Factors other than disease
- Operating characteristics
- Sensitivity and specificity
- Prevalence of disease in the population
The reasons why tests rarely give a yes/no answer are outlined in this chapter.

## Normal values

Most test results are expressed as continuous variables therefore there is an overlap between test results in patients who have and do not have a disease. However, it is necessary to define a cut-off point at which the test is said to be normal or abnormal. This cut-off point is chosen to minimise the number of false positives and false negatives. With any normal distribution, there are people whose test results lie at the extremes, but that does not mean they have a disease (see Figure 3.1). In the figure, moving the cut-off point to the right would increase the chance of picking up 'abnormals' but at the same time increase the rate of false positives. This is always a trade-off in diagnostic tests.

Arbitrarily dividing a *range* of values into 'normal' and 'abnormal' has disadvantages – it does not take into account the magnitude of the result. For example, a highly sensitive troponin T result in a patient with chest pain is more likely to indicate a myocardial infarction when the value is very high, as opposed to slightly raised.

In medicine there are some situations when a normal result is abnormal, and an abnormal result is normal – for example in a clinically severe asthma attack when one expects the $PaCO_2$ to be low, a normal $PaCO_2$ indicates life-threatening asthma. On the other hand, a low serum ferritin is considered normal in young menstruating women. Therefore, even 'normal' and 'abnormal' values have to be interpreted by a clinician.

## Factors other than disease that influence test results

A number of factors other than disease influence test results, such as:
- Age
- Sex
- Ethnicity
- Pregnancy
- Body position
- Chance
- Spurious (*in vitro*) results
- Lab error
For example, normal values for paediatric blood results are often significantly different to those for adults. Old people commonly have a normal white cell count in sepsis, and can have a

---

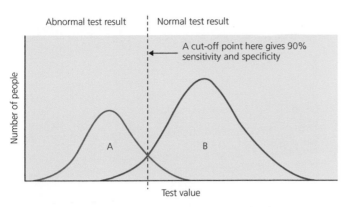

**Figure 3.1** Distribution of results in people with (A) and without (B) a disease.

significantly reduced glomerular filtration rate with a normal creatinine. Men have slightly different values from women (e.g. for haemoglobin), and young black men may have an 'abnormal' 12-lead electrocardiogram (a so-called 'normal variant').

Pregnancy significantly alters many test results due to physiological changes that occur, particularly in the third trimester. A large foetus splints the diaphragm and compresses the lungs causing supine hypoxaemia as well as a respiratory alkalosis (important facts to remember when considering the possibility of a pulmonary embolism in a pregnant woman). Circulating volume increases by 50% in late pregnancy causing a flow murmur, tachycardia and a rightward axis on the 12-lead electrocardiogram. Kidneys also swell as a result, and renal ultrasound shows increased size and dilatation.

Body position is important in some tests, for example lung function, and tests where the patient has to lie in a certain position to get optimal images. Finally, a test result may be abnormal by chance (i.e. the patient is an outlier on the normal curve); the result may be spurious (e.g. hyperkalaemia caused by haemolysis or some haematological conditions); or may be due to lab error (e.g. as a result of technical or human failure). It is always worth pausing before acting when an unexpected test result crops up.

## Operating characteristics

Before ordering a test, it is important to be aware of certain operating characteristics of the test. This refers to the method of performing the test. For example, measuring lung function requires that the patient be able to hear, understand and co-operate with instructions, as well as hold their breath. Exercise electrocardiograms are inappropriate in patients who have left bundle branch block or who cannot walk.

Some tests, for example in ultrasound and echocardiography, are 'operator dependent' – that is, the skill of the operator influences the results and the report provided. Others are influenced by the patient's body habitus or anatomy. If a report says, 'Limited views due to…' then it is important to note that an abnormality may not have been excluded.

Some conditions are paroxysmal. In epilepsy, 50% of patients have a normal electroencephalogram (EEG) between attacks. Syncope is another good example of a paroxysmal condition

where diagnostic testing is only able to gather circumstantial evidence. These two conditions are mainly diagnosed on the history given by the patient and an eyewitness. On the other hand, up to 10% of normal people have epileptiform discharges on an EEG but they do not have epilepsy – this is known as an incidental finding and does not mean the patient has a disease at all. 'Incidentalomas' are common findings in computed tomography (CT) reports.

## Sensitivity and specificity

Sensitivity is the ability of a test to detect true positives, whereas specificity is the ability to detect true negatives. Unfortunately, there is no such thing as a perfect test. Nearly all tests have less than 100% sensitivity and specificity. Therefore, there are 'true positives' and 'false positives', 'true negatives' and 'false negatives'. Table 3.1 illustrates this. Tests differ from each other in sensitivity and specificity for detecting certain diseases, and clinicians need to have a rough idea how good a test is for the disease under investigation.

A very sensitive test will detect most diseases but also generate abnormal results in healthy people. A positive result is therefore likely to require further evaluation. On the other hand, a very specific test will miss diseases but is more likely to establish the diagnosis when the result is positive.

In simple terms, the probability that a patient has a disease depends on the clinical (pre-test) probability plus the sensitivity and the specificity of the test. The clinical probability of a disease is assessed *mainly by listening to the patient's story*, combined with the clinician's knowledge of epidemiology and medicine. For example, the clinical probability of a 60-year-old male smoker with diabetes who presents with dull, central chest pain radiating to his jaw on exertion having coronary artery disease is high. This is the termed the pre-test or prior probability. Post-test or posterior probability is the probability of the disease after acquiring new information using tests. In medicine we estimate post-test probability all the time. What we are dealing with is something called conditional probability.

Conditional probability is the probability that something is true given that something else is true. For example, a patient presents with chest pain. He has a normal 12-lead electrocardiogram. His highly sensitive troponin T result is slightly raised. What is the probability of a heart attack in this patient? The answer is not as obvious as it seems. To start with, more information about the patient is required so that his clinical (pre-test) probability can be estimated.

**Table 3.1** Sensitivity and specificity. Sensitivity is the probability that the test will indicate disease in those *with* the disease, i.e. $A/(A+C) \times 100$. Specificity is the probability that the test will be negative in those without the disease, i.e. $D/(D+B) \times 100$.

|  | Disease | No disease |
| --- | --- | --- |
| Positive test | A (True positive) | B (False positive) |
| Negative test | C (False negative) | D (True negative) |

Box 3.1 **How a test results shifts our thinking from an initial impression to a final impression, using Bayes' theorem.**

The sensitivity of a troponin test is 95% and the specificity is 80%. If we imagine a patient with chest pain and our pre-test or prior probability is 50% (i.e. we are sitting on the fence), this is how a positive or a negative result would shift our thinking about whether the patient is having a heart attack. As clinicians become more expert, their probability estimates become more accurate.

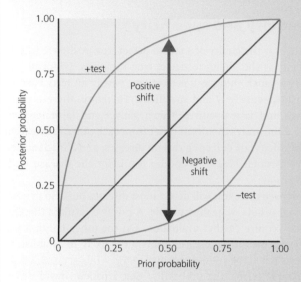

Bayes' theorem is a method for interpreting evidence in the context of previous knowledge. It has wide applications and constitutes a mathematical foundation for reasoning. In clinical practice, doctors do not use algebra to work out pre- and post-test probabilities; however, an understanding of the principles of Bayes' theorem ('Bayesian reasoning') is important because the ability to accurately estimate probability is a hallmark of a good clinician and our intuitive estimates of probability are often inaccurate.

Bayes' theorem:

$$P[Dis/R+] = \frac{P[R+/Dis] \times P[Dis]}{P[R+/Dis] \times P[Dis] + P[R+/no\ Dis] \times P[no\ Dis]}$$

where P[Dis/R+] is the chance of having the disease given a positive test result, and P is probability, Dis is disease and R+ is a positive test result.

Figure from Brush JE. Probability: uncertainty quantified. In: *The Science of the Art of Medicine*, 2015. Reproduced with permission of Dementi Milestone Publishing.

Bayes' theorem (named after English clergyman Thomas Bayes 1702–61) is a mathematical way to describe the post-test or posterior probability of a disease. It gives a way to shift our thinking from an initial impression to a final impression, based on a positive or negative test result. It incorporates the sensitivity and specificity of the test with our initial clinical (pre-test) probability estimate. Box 3.1 illustrates Bayes' theorem further and a more detailed explanation can be found in 'Further reading/resources'.

For patients with very low or very high clinical probabilities, a test result has less effect on post-test probability, and you should

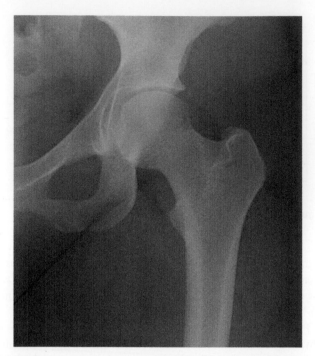

**Figure 3.2** A 70-year-old woman was admitted following a fall. She had hurt her left hip and was unable to weight bear. On examination, the left leg was externally rotated and extremely painful to move. Is there a fracture?

consider in some circumstances whether to do the test at all. A common misconception among both clinicians and patients is to think that a test result gives the answer.

Figure 3.2 illustrates a common clinical dilemma. Both anteroposterior and lateral views of the left hip are required, and in this case they are normal. But clinically there seems to be a high probability of a fracture. Because the probability of a disease depends on the clinical (pre-test) probability as well as the sensitivity and the specificity of the test, a normal X-ray cannot exclude a fracture in a high clinical probability patient. On the other hand, the combination of a low clinical probability and a normal X-ray *would* exclude a fracture. The same test result is interpreted completely differently when the clinical (pre-test) probability changes. The lesson from these examples is that tests, even good tests, might be wrong.

The correct use of tests is even more important when the test is very sensitive but not very specific, or vice versa. D-dimer is a very sensitive test for pulmonary thromboembolism (98% sensitivity), but not very specific (40% specificity). With a high pre-test probability a negative D-dimer still leaves a chance of a pulmonary embolism. With a low pre-test probability, a negative D-dimer virtually excludes the diagnosis. D-dimer is a good example of a commonly misunderstood and misused test.

## Prevalence of disease in the population

Consider this problem that was given to a group of Harvard doctors: if a test to detect a disease whose prevalence is 1:1000 has a false positive rate of 5%, what is the chance that a person found to have a positive result actually has the disease, assuming you know nothing about the person's symptoms or signs? Just under half replied with the answer 95%. Now look at Box 3.2 for the answer.

Box 3.2 **What is the chance a person found to have a positive result actually has the disease?**

Many doctors answer this question intuitively, giving an answer of 95% (using 'type 1 thinking', which is explained further in Chapter 4) but the real answer is illustrated in the table below:

|  | Disease | No disease | Total |
|---|---|---|---|
| Actual | 1 | 999 | 1000 |
| Positive test | 1 | 50 | 51 |
| Negative test | 0 | 949 | 949 |

The question tells us that 50/1000 people will have a false positive result. But only 1/1000 has the disease. This means the chance of having a positive result *and* actually having the disease is 1 out of 51 – or 2%. This example illustrates the importance of understanding prevalence (or the denominator in probability terms).

Box 3.3 **Predictive values**

|  | Disease | No disease |
|---|---|---|
| Positive test | A<br>(True positive) | B<br>(False positive) |
| Negative test | C<br>(False negative) | D<br>(True negative) |

The positive predictive value – 'what is the chance that a person with a positive test truly has the disease?' – is A/(A+B)×100. The negative predictive value is D/(D+C)×100.

Positive and negative predictive values are influenced by the prevalence of the disease in the population being tested. Using a test in a population with higher prevalence increases positive predictive value (and decreases negative predictive value).

Box 3.4 **Interpreting test results**

Results of imaging stress testing in a 35-year-old woman with non-cardiac sounding chest pain (Table A) and a 65-year-old man with typical symptoms of angina (Table B). IHD = ischaemic heart disease.

**Table A**

|  | IHD | No IHD |
|---|---|---|
| Actual/total | 1 | 99 |
| Positive test | 0.9<br>True positive (sensitivity) | 14.9 |
| Negative test | 0.1 | 84.1<br>True negative (specificity) |

**Table B**

|  | IHD | No IHD |
|---|---|---|
| Actual/total | 94 | 6 |
| Positive test | 84.6<br>True positive (sensitivity) | 0.9 |
| Negative test | 9.4 | 5.1<br>True negative (specificity) |

Although both patients had some kind of chest pain and both were sent for the same test, how we interpret a positive result is completely different for each one. In the young woman's case the clinical probability and prevalence of disease is low and therefore a positive imaging stress test result is 15 times more likely to be wrong than right. In the older man, however, the opposite is true – a negative test should be viewed with suspicion because it is twice as likely to be wrong than right. The same test result in a completely different patient has to be interpreted completely differently.

The prevalence of the disease in the population has an impact on the interpretation of a test result. *Predictive values* are the combination of sensitivity, specificity and prevalence. Sensitivity and specificity are characteristics of the test. The population does not affect the result. But as clinicians, we are interested in whether a person with a positive test result truly has the disease. Box 3.3 illustrates predictive values.

John Brush, in his book *The Science of the Art of Medicine* (see 'Further reading/resources'), uses this example to illustrate. We know from angiography results and post-mortem studies the actual prevalence of coronary artery disease in different patient groups. Young women with non-cardiac sounding chest pain have a low prevalence of ischaemic heart disease. On the other hand, older men with typical symptoms of angina have a high prevalence of ischaemic heart disease. If we sent a patient from each of these groups for an imaging stress test, and both tests came back positive, how would we interpret the results?

On average, an imaging stress test has a sensitivity of 90% and a specificity of 85%. The actual prevalence of ischaemic heart disease in a young woman (aged 35 years) with non-cardiac sounding chest pain is around 1% but the prevalence of ischaemic heart disease in an older man (aged 65 years) with typical symptoms of angina is around 94% – that is a huge difference. Aside from the fact that we should consider whether to request this test at all in patients with such extreme pre-test probabilities, Box 3.4 shows the results we would get if we tested 100 patients just like them.

This example illustrates the problems that can be encountered when clinicians use tests without considering the predictive value of the test for the individual patient. Boxes 3.5 and 3.6 give further clinical examples.

## Thresholds

An important consideration in the diagnostic process is whether to do a test at all. If a test will make no difference to the probability or outcome of a disease, should the test be done? Tests are most helpful when they change the management of a patient's condition.

The *therapeutic threshold* combines factors such as test characteristics, risks of the test, availability, and the risks versus benefits of treatment. The point at which the factors are all evenly weighed is the threshold. If a test or treatment for a disease is effective and low risk then one would have a lower threshold for going ahead.

### Box 3.5 **Thinking about tests – D-dimer**

A 25 year-old-man with no risk factors for venous thromboembolism went to see his general practitioner (GP) with pleuritic-sounding chest pain. He gave a clear description of doing some building work and pulling a muscle two days before, but he made the appointment as the pain was not controlled with simple painkillers. The patient had a past medical history of Crohn's disease and was taking medication for this. He was otherwise fit and well. Although the GP felt pulmonary embolism was unlikely, he requested a D-dimer test *to exclude it.* The result was 625 ng/mL (normal <500 ng/mL) and so the patient was admitted to hospital for further evaluation. He was scheduled by a junior doctor for a CT pulmonary angiogram.

*What would you do in this situation?*

D-dimer has a sensitivity of around 98% and a specificity of around 40%. This means it is nearly always raised when venous thromboembolism is present but not necessarily normal when venous thromboembolism is absent. D-dimer can be raised for lots of other reasons that have nothing to do with venous thromboembolism (including muscle tears and inflammatory bowel disease). The starting point for using a D-dimer test is when you think, on the basis of the history and examination, a patient has venous thromboembolism. It is useful in virtually excluding low clinical probability patients who then do not need to go on to have further tests. This is *different* to requesting a D-dimer in a patient whose history clearly points to chest pain from another cause.

### Box 3.6 **Thinking about tests – CT head**

A 74-year-old woman with a past medical history of hypertension attended the Emergency Department because of sudden weakness of her left leg. She was able to walk. Mild weakness was confirmed on clinical examination. A doctor ordered a CT scan of the head to look for a stroke and informed the patient of his suspicion. Her CT head was normal. Subsequently, the doctor told the patient that she had *not* had a stroke, reassured her and discharged her from the Emergency Department.

*What would you do in this situation?*

Stroke is a clinical diagnosis and the CT head is often normal in stroke. This doctor made the mistake of believing that the test, rather than the history and examination, made the diagnosis in this situation.

On the other hand, if a test or treatment is less effective or high risk, one requires greater confidence in the clinical diagnosis and potential benefits of treatment first. Box 3.7 illustrates thresholds, using suspected acute appendicitis as an example.

### Box 3.7 **Thresholds – for example in suspected acute appendicitis**

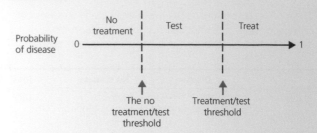

- If the diagnosis of appendicitis is clear from the history and examination, treatment without further testing is indicated.
- When the diagnosis of appendicitis is uncertain, the use of computed tomography (CT) scanning can aid in diagnosis and reduce the risk of perforation.
- The Alvarado score is a useful diagnostic 'rule out' score in suspected appendicitis, helping to identify those patients who can be observed without treatment. Using guidelines, scores and decision aids is described further in Chapter 8.

## Summary

Tests do not make a diagnosis, clinicians do (unfortunately, patients do not necessarily understand this when they ask, 'What do the test results show?'). *Tests give us test probabilities not real probabilities.* Tests should be requested rationally and the results have to be interpreted. Assessing clinical (pre-test) probability is vital. Without it, you cannot interpret any test result. A working knowledge of factors other than disease that influence test results, operating characteristic and how good the test is for the disease in question is also important. The predictive value of a test result not only depends on the test's sensitivity and specificity, but also on the prevalence of the disease in the population in question. Thresholds provide a useful way of thinking about whether a test should be performed at all.

## Further reading/resources

Brush JE. *The Science of the Art of Medicine.* Dementi Milestone Publishing, 2015.

Ohle R, O'Reilly F, O'Brien K et al. The Alvarado Score for predicting acute appendicitis: a systematic review. *BMC Medicine* 2011; **9**:139. Available at: www.biomedcentral.com/1741-7015/9/139 (accessed 15 February 2016).

Royal College of Physicians of London. *Doctors in Society. Medical Professionalism in a Changing World.* London: RCP, 2005.

Sox HC, Higgins MC, Owens DK. *Medical Decision Making*, 2nd edn. Oxford: Wiley-Blackwell, 2013.

Stone JV. *Bayes' Rule. A tutorial introduction to Bayesian analysis.* Sebtel Press, 2013.

# CHAPTER 4

# Models of Clinical Reasoning

*Martin Hughes[1] and Graham Nimmo[2]*

[1] Royal Infirmary, Glasgow, UK
[2] Western General Hospital, Edinburgh, UK

## OVERVIEW

- Clinical reasoning is complex and incompletely understood
- Dual process theory divides thinking into intuitive (type 1) and analytical (type 2) thinking
- We use various types of reasoning in assorted circumstances
- There are several reasons why faulty reasoning occurs
- Experts and novices reason differently

## Introduction

Reasoning is the process of using existing knowledge to draw conclusions, make predictions, or construct explanations. Clinical reasoning involves diagnosis and decisions about further diagnostic tests and treatment.

In this chapter, we will explain different types of reasoning, consider dual process theory (type 1 and type 2 thinking), and explore the advantages and disadvantages of each. We will look at types of errors that occur in the reasoning process, and will also compare the approaches of experts to those of novices.

It is important to be aware that research in the area of clinical reasoning can be artificial and tends to produce different behaviours and cognitive processes than is probably the case normally (the Hawthorne effect). For example, speaking out loud about your thought processes, a common research method, is not the same as thinking without speaking. Knowing that your thinking is being analysed is likely to make you take additional time and second guess yourself more. Importantly, most research concerns type 2 thinking rather than the much more prevalent type 1 thinking.

Although we can differentiate some of the ways experienced clinicians and inexperienced novices reason, what we really desire as an outcome is for every experienced clinician to be excellent. Unfortunately not all experienced clinicians perform to the same high standard. Until we can find a way to differentiate outstanding from average, and distinguish the way that outstanding clinicians reason, the goal of excellence for every experienced clinician may be unattainable.

## Deductive reasoning

Box 4.1 lists the different types of reasoning used in clinical practice.

Deductive reasoning starts with a general rule and moves towards a specific conclusion. If the original premises are true, the conclusion must also be true. For example:
- Premise 1: Anaemia is a haemoglobin below the normal value
- Premise 2: Mrs Smith has a haemoglobin below the normal value
- Conclusion: Mrs Smith is anaemic

The conclusion of a deductive argument may be sound or unsound, depending on whether the premises are true. However, the deductive inference itself may still be valid even if the premises are nonsense. For example:
- Premise 1: Anaemia is a sodium concentration of less than 120 mmol/L
- Premise 2: Mrs Smith has a sodium concentration of less than 120 mmol/L
- Conclusion: Mrs Smith is anaemic

This is *unsound* because the first premise is false, but logically *valid*, because if the premises were true the conclusion would also be true. The advantage of deductive reasoning is the absolute certainty of conclusions reached if the premises are true. However, it is impossible to make predictions about unknown future events.

## Hypothetico-deductive reasoning

Hypothetico-deductive reasoning is one of the strategies that clinicians employ to make a diagnosis. A hypothesis is generated and arguments made, for example:
- Premise 1: In Disease A, finding B occurs
- Premise 2: B is absent
- Conclusion: Disease A is not the diagnosis

The disadvantages of this type of 'detective work' are two-fold. Normally, this deduction can only rule out some of the possibilities and a definite conclusion cannot be reached. Occasionally, only one diagnostic possibility will remain after excluding other hypotheses and the diagnosis is made. But we

*ABC of Clinical Reasoning*, First Edition. Edited by Nicola Cooper and John Frain.
© 2017 John Wiley & Sons, Ltd. Published 2017 by John Wiley & Sons, Ltd.

Box 4.1 **Types of reasoning**

- Deduction
- Induction
- Abduction
- Rule-based/categorical/deterministic
- Probabilistic
- Type 1
- Type 2

Box 4.2 **Mr Jones' abdominal pain – deduction**

Mr Jones, who has gallstones, presented with a short history of upper abdominal pain. As part of the investigations, after we have come to the conclusion that the most likely diagnosis is acute cholecystitis (see below), a serum amylase is ordered. We can formally state this logic:

*Deduction 1*

- Premise 1: Patients presenting with acute severe upper abdominal pain should have a serum amylase measured as part of a complete assessment
- Premise 2: Mr Jones has acute severe upper abdominal pain
- Conclusion: I will check serum amylase

To reach the conclusion we are using deduction.

*Deduction 2*

- Premise 1: In disease A, finding B occurs – in biliary obstruction due to gallstones, jaundice is present
- Premise 2: B is absent – jaundice is absent
- Conclusion: Disease A is not the diagnosis – biliary obstruction is not the diagnosis

Box 4.3 **Mr Jones' abdominal pain – induction**

- Evidence: Mr Jones has vomited blood. His haemoglobin Hb is 73 g/L. He is hypotensive and tachycardic. He has recently been complaining of epigastric pain and had an oesophago-gastro-duodenoscopy, which showed a gastric ulcer.
- Conclusion: We are reasonably certain that Mr Smith has a bleeding gastric ulcer.

cannot be certain that we have considered, and therefore excluded, every competing hypothesis.

Deductive reasoning is commonly used in medicine, but its use is generally subconscious (see Box 4.2). It allows us to organise our thinking using rules, background knowledge and hypotheses to reach a conclusion.

## Inductive reasoning

In inductive reasoning we move from specific observations to a more general conclusion (the opposite of deduction). Science and medicine rely heavily on inductive reasoning. We gather evidence, seek patterns, and form a hypothesis or theory to explain what is seen. We have evidence (A), leading to conclusions (B) – see Box 4.3.

The conclusions reached by inductive reasoning are only probable, not guaranteed. No amount of evidence makes an

Box 4.4 **Mr Jones' abdominal pain – abduction**

- Mr Jones has vomited blood. His haemoglobin is 73 g/L. He is hypotensive and tachycardic.
- We have no other history.
- The most likely cause (our best guess) is bleeding from his upper gastro-intestinal tract.

Endoscopy may reveal a gastric ulcer, or varices, or a tumour or an aorto-duodenal fistula. The history might be wrong, and it was actually haemoptysis; or the blood is a red herring, and he has developed septic shock due to an unrelated infection...

**Table 4.1** Rule-based/categorical/deterministic reasoning.

| Familiar problem | Routine |
|---|---|
| Middle-aged female with dysuria, frequency and urgency | Urine culture and treat for a urinary tract infection |
| Fever and inflammatory response in a patient recently treated for pneumonia | Chest X-ray – consider an empyema or lung abscess |
| Hyponatraemia | Assess volume status, measure serum and urine electrolytes and osmolalities, thyroid and liver function tests and cortisol |

inductive conclusion certain. We do not know whether all of the evidence has been gathered, or if a further piece of evidence may arise to invalidate the conclusion.

Inductive arguments are described as either *cogent* (the evidence seems comprehensive, it is pertinent, and generally credible) or *not cogent*, rather than being true or untrue. Inductive reasoning allows prediction of future, or previously unobserved, events.

## Abductive reasoning

Often in the real world we cannot form a good deductive argument, nor a convincing (cogent) inductive one. Here, we tend to use abductive reasoning – working backwards from signs, symptoms and investigations to causes; that is, from effect to cause rather from cause to effect. It is similar to inductive reasoning in that it is inherently uncertain. Abduction is a process of choosing the hypothesis that would best explain the available evidence. We ask ourselves, 'What is the likeliest answer?' 'What theory best explains this information?' We have information (B) and move backwards to likely cause (A) – see Box 4.4.

## Rule-based/categorical/deterministic reasoning

During day-to-day clinical encounters much of our reasoning is relatively simple, at least when we encounter familiar problems. We have an established set of routines that we use on a regular basis. Table 4.1 shows an example.

Novices will struggle with this type of approach because they do not have the necessary experience and knowledge to have compiled a database of standard responses, and experts acting outside their area of expertise will similarly be unable to resort to this method.

## Probabilistic reasoning

Probabilistic reasoning is the clinician's substitute for formal Bayesian analysis (described in Chapter 3). Doctors use probabilistic reasoning in many situations – we are thinking consciously but are often unaware we are using estimated base rates (e.g. chest infections are very common) and then conditional probabilities (e.g. negative sputum culture result) to modify hypotheses. Unfortunately, even for simple investigations with known pre-test and conditional probabilities, the estimates given by doctors for post-test probabilities are very inaccurate.

Probabilistic reasoning is used to classify the likelihood of the hypotheses we generate, and to modify these hypotheses when the results of tests are known. The probabilities we use are not normally based on good information, but on the clinician's knowledge and experience of the conditions, and the interpretation of the usefulness of tests to change the likelihood of a disease. Knowledge of Bayesian analysis, pre-test probabilities and likelihood ratios for the tests we use may improve our accuracy and the usefulness of probabilistic reasoning.

## Causal reasoning

In causal reasoning, clinicians use their knowledge of medical sciences to provide additional diagnostic information. For example, if considering thyrotoxicosis as a diagnosis, a raised thyroxine would be expected, but so would a suppressed thyroid stimulating hormone (TSH). In the absence of this confirmatory finding, other diagnostic possibilities must be considered (e.g. 'sick euthyroid').

Causal reasoning is normally used to confirm or refute hypotheses generated using other reasoning strategies. It is not particularly helpful by itself in producing a hypothesis.

## Making a diagnosis – hypothesis generation and modification

Using deduction, induction/abduction, rule-based reasoning, or mental short cuts (heuristics), clinicians come up with a hypothesis, or hypotheses, which may be specific (pneumonia or pulmonary embolus) or general (infection or inflammation), relating a specific situation to knowledge and past experience. This process is referred to as generating a differential diagnosis.

The process we use to produce a differential diagnosis from memory is not clear. The new facts of the case may be compared to a disease prototype built over years, adding gradually to the variations and different presentations we might expect. The hypotheses chosen may be based on likelihood, but might also reflect the need to rule out the worst case scenario, even if the probability is considered low. We regularly use heuristics (like availability, representativeness, life-threatening condition).

Hypothesis generation is often not perfect, and rare diseases, or those with atypical features, may never be thought of. It is the earliest stage of diagnosis where knowledge deficits and cognitive biases (see Chapter 5) may lead to errors. Hypothesis generation is the first part of *iterative* diagnosis, or what has traditionally

**Table 4.2** Type 1 and type 2 thinking – dual process theory.

| Type 1 thinking | Type 2 thinking |
| --- | --- |
| • Intuitive, uses mental shortcuts (heuristics) | • Analytical, systematic |
| • Automatic, subconscious | • Deliberate, conscious |
| • Fast, effortless | • Slow, effortful |
| • Low/variable reliability | • High/consistent reliability |
| • Vulnerable to error | • Less prone to error |
| • Highly affected by context | • Less affected by context |
| • High emotional involvement | • Low emotional involvement |
| • Low scientific rigour | • High scientific rigour |

been referred to as *hypothetico-deductive reasoning*. A different way to think about this process is to consider it one of *hypothesis modification*.

Hypothesis modification aims to produce a working diagnosis: is each theory coherent, sufficient and parsimonious? Hypotheses are often generated quickly and may be discarded equally quickly. Only a few can remain active at any one time due to the limitations of short-term memory. We gather information within the context of a hypothesis, or a set of hypotheses, rather than just accumulating information blindly. The modification process may be short and sharp for cases that are typical, straightforward or within our area of expertise. It may be more prolonged and detailed for complicated or unfamiliar cases. We can try to *confirm* or *disconfirm,* and when we have two closely related hypotheses we attempt to *discriminate*.

Hypothesis refinement uses probabilistic, causal and rule-based (categorical) reasoning. It uses investigations to test theories (hypothetico-deduction). Depending on the case, the information available, and the clinician's knowledge and experience, the working diagnosis will be formulated using any one of the different types of reasoning, or more commonly a combination of more than one.

The diagnosis may be clear and unambiguous or we may need more abduction: what is the best option available, and are we confident enough to make a decision on treatment, or can we wait?

## Type 1 and type 2 thinking – dual process theory

Cognitive psychology deals with human thinking, reasoning and decision-making. Dual process theory describes how the human brain has two distinct 'minds' when it comes to decision-making. There are forms of cognition that are ancient and shared with other animals – where speed is often more important than accuracy – and ones that are recently evolved and distinctly human. Each 'mind' has access to multiple systems in the brain. We have a fast, pattern recognising, intuitive way of thinking (type 1); and a slow, controlled but high effort way of thinking (type 2) – see Table 4.2.

We spend most of our lives in type 1 mode and clinicians are no exception. Imagine the cognitive effort involved in learning to drive a car, for example. We could not live our lives permanently in a deliberate, slow, effortful way. Over time driving becomes automatic and subconscious. In the same way, a lot of our clinical decision-making is intuitive rather than analytical. But it is not an either/or

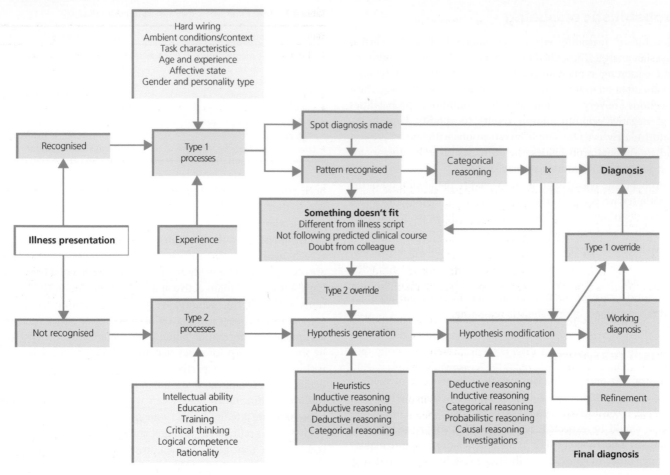

**Figure 4.1** A modified universal model of diagnostic reasoning. Although type 1 processes are intuitive, it does not mean that the decision-maker is unaware of them or that they cannot be changed. A clinician can pause to check his or her thinking and assumptions at any time. This 'type 2 override' (sometimes called 'rational override') is often triggered when something doesn't fit, leading to thinking about things more analytically. In the same way, clinicians sometimes use 'type 1 override' (or 'irrational override' – although it is not always bad) – an example would be overriding a validated scoring system, for example the revised Geneva score for pulmonary embolism, which consistently outperforms clinical judgement, and despite a low score and negative D-dimer requesting a CT pulmonary angiogram anyway on the basis of 'gut feeling'. Ix = investigations.

situation. We can pause to analyse what we are doing. We can also actively switch between between one type of thinking and the other if we understand which type of thinking we are engaged in.

For example, imagine going to see a drowsy patient in the Emergency Department. He is known to have alcohol dependence and is a frequent attender. The problem is recognised and familiar. It would be easy to *assume* you know what the problem is. In a well-calibrated thinker, this is when analytical thinking comes into play, as illustrated in Figure 4.1.

Figure 4.1 shows a modified version of Croskerry's 'Universal Model of Diagnostic Reasoning'. Building on this, we have developed some changes that more clearly delineate the processes clinicians use on a daily basis.

As in Croskerry's model, we may recognise the problem at hand. It could be as simple as a spot diagnosis (e.g. shingles) or it could lead to simple rule-based reactions that over the years have become automatic (as in Table 4.1). However, if the problem is unrecognised, the first stage in the diagnostic process is hypothesis generation, or formation of a differential diagnosis, as described above. Hypothesis modification will proceed

until there is enough certainty for a *working diagnosis*. The degree of certainty required will depend on the treatment needed – for example, the diagnosis of a simple urinary tract infection does not need the same degree of certainty as a diagnosis of leukaemia before treatment is commenced. Similarly with the investigations – a urine sample requires a lower level of suspicion for a urinary tract infection than a bone marrow aspirate does for leukaemia. Further diagnostic refinement is often required (what type of leukaemia is it; what organism is causing the urine infection?) before a final diagnosis is reached, or the hypothesis changed.

## Errors in the diagnostic process

There are five types of error in the diagnostic process:
- No fault errors
- System errors
- Errors due to knowledge gaps
- Errors due to misinterpretation of diagnostic tests
- Cognitive errors

Box 4.5 **Examples of system errors leading to errors in the diagnostic process**

- Inadequate staffing
- Lack of senior supervision
- Poor working conditions
- Lack of diagnostic facilities
- Poor information technology and reference facilities
- Deficient lines of communication

These conditions form the context in which a decision is made.

No fault errors are ones in which no clinician could have made the diagnosis – the history was unavailable, the patient withheld information or the presentation was so atypical it could not be recognised. Examples of system errors are illustrated in Box 4.5. Knowledge gaps are an important factor in diagnostic errors – no amount of brilliant reasoning will trigger a diagnostic hypothesis if the clinician is unaware of a disease, or a specific manifestation of a disease.

Tests are commonly misused by clinicians. We do not understand the information we receive from tests. Tests change the probabilities of a particular disease being present or absent, but rarely in a binary yes/no fashion – this is discussed in more detail in Chapter 3.

Finally, cognitive errors are subconscious errors in our thinking processes. These account for the majority of fundamental causes of diagnostic error. Some common examples are listed in Table 4.3. Cognitive errors may occur at any stage during the reasoning process and, while they are most strongly associated with type 1 thinking, they also occur in type 2 thinking.

## The reasoning of experts versus novices

There do appear to be differences in the reasoning strategies used by novices compared with those used by experts. In their particular subject matter domain, experts use very purposeful information gathering, with strongly effective problem-solving strategies. Heuristics are commonly, and most often successfully, used. The expert will have a saved bank of illness scripts with which to compare and contrast the current case. Overall, they will use type 1 thinking more than the novice, and with much better results.

In order to become an expert one needs specific knowledge and specific experience. The very nature of being a novice means they have little experience with the problems they face, and have not built a bank of illness scripts, and will have no memories of previous similar cases or of their previous actions in such cases. Therefore their search strategies will be weak, slow and ponderous. They will consider a far wider range of diagnostic possibilities and will take longer to select approaches to discriminate among them.

Moving from novice to expert in medicine has traditionally been achieved by gradually gaining experience while observing the reasoning of experts – 'learning by osmosis'. It seems likely that explicit teaching of clinical reasoning could make this process

**Table 4.3** Some common cognitive errors in medicine.

| Bias | Description |
| --- | --- |
| Anchoring | Having latched onto a particular aspect of the initial consultation, we refuse to change our mind about the importance of the aspect |
| Confirmation bias | Once we have made an initial diagnosis, we tend to accept evidence that backs our hypothesis and ignore evidence that refutes it |
| Premature closure | We make a diagnosis before all the information has been gathered or verified. This involves short-cutting to the final diagnosis stage when we should only be at the hypotheses generation and modification stage |
| Search satisficing | Once we have made a diagnosis, we forget that there may be others. We commonly miss second fractures, or second poisoning agents |
| Posterior probability error | Short-cutting to the patient's usual diagnosis. He may have presented with confusion and agitation from alcohol withdrawal many times before, but it is wise to check for alternatives, such as pneumonia or subdural haematoma |
| Outcome bias | Our desire for a certain outcome alters our judgement (e.g. a surgeon blaming sepsis on pneumonia rather than an anastomotic leak) |

quicker, and more effective, but there is little evidence currently to support this proposition.

## Summary

Clinical reasoning is complex – it often requires various mental processes operating simultaneously during the same clinical encounter, as well as different processes for different situations. These mental processes can be described in different ways, as in Box 4.1. Dual process theory describes how humans have two distinct approaches when it comes to decision-making. We have a fast, pattern recognising, intuitive way of thinking (type 1); and a slow, controlled but high effort way of thinking (type 2). In everyday life, we spend most of our time in type 1 mode. However, our thinking is frequently flawed. There are numerous causes for failure in clinical reasoning and these can occur in any type of reasoning and at any stage in the process. While experts and novices reason differently, even experts are liable to subconscious errors in their thinking processes – an area explored in more detail in the next chapter.

## Further reading/resources

Croskerry P. A universal model of diagnostic reasoning. *Acad Med* 2009; **84**:1–7.

Graber M, Franklin N, Gordon R. Diagnostic error in internal medicine. *Arch Intern Med* 2005; **165**:1493–9.

Hughes M, Nimmo G. Communication and decision-making in intensive care. In: Nimmo G and Singer M (eds), *ABC of Intensive Care*, 2nd edn. Wiley-Blackwell, Oxford, 2011.

Kassirer J, Wong J, Kopelman R. *Learning Clinical Reasoning*. Lippincott Williams & Wilkins, 2010.

Norman GR, Eva KW. Diagnostic error and clinical reasoning. *Med Educ* 2010: **44**:94–100.

# CHAPTER 5

# Cognitive Biases

*Nicola Cooper*

Derby Teaching Hospitals NHS Foundation Trust; and University of Nottingham, UK

---

> **OVERVIEW**
> - Cognitive biases are prevalent in everyday thinking and healthcare professionals are no exception
> - Cognitive biases play an important role in diagnostic error
> - Some common cognitive biases applicable to healthcare are described here
> - Cognitive errors are not only the preserve of type 1 thinking
> - Cognitive biases should not be confused with expert intuition, which plays an important role in expert professional practice

## Introduction

Medical education emphasises knowledge and clinical skills but little attention has been given to teaching students and trainees about thinking itself. Chapter 4 explored models of clinical reasoning, including dual process theory. Psychologists reckon we spend 95% of our time in type 1 mode – the intuitive, pattern recognising, effortless mode of thinking. But the price we pay for this low-resource mode of decision-making is bias – or, to use a less negative term, *cognitive dispositions to respond*. Bias, or our tendency to respond in certain ways, is so widespread that 'we need to consider it as a normal operating characteristic of the brain' (see 'Further reading/resources'). Humans are quite irrational at times, and healthcare professionals are no exception.

In his book *The Art of Thinking Clearly*, Dobelli describes 99 cognitive biases prevalent in everyday life, ranging from 'sunk cost fallacy' to 'confirmation bias' to 'neglect of probability' to 'decision fatigue'. Many of these are particularly applicable to healthcare. He writes, 'In the 1960s, psychologists began to examine our thinking, decisions and actions scientifically. The result was a theory of irrationality: thinking itself is not pure, but prone to error. This affects everyone. Even highly intelligent people fall in to the same cognitive traps. Likewise, errors are not randomly distributed. We systematically err in the same direction. That makes our mistakes predictable, and thus fixable to some degree – but only to a degree, never completely.'

This chapter is about the different cognitive biases we are all prone to, in our everyday lives and as healthcare professionals. The next chapter on human factors explores the limitations of human performance further.

## Case history

A 75-year-old woman presented to hospital with breathlessness. She had been told by her oncologist a few weeks before that she was anaemic, and to report to hospital if she got breathless or dizzy in case she needed a blood transfusion. Her haemoglobin at presentation was 84 g/L, which was unchanged from previously. Her only past medical history was breast cancer for which she had had a mastectomy and was undergoing adjuvant chemotherapy. She was usually fit and independent and was not taking any regular medication apart from anti-emetics.

On examination, the chest, heart and abdomen were normal. Her vital signs were normal. Her 12-lead electrocardiogram was normal. Apart from the haemoglobin of 84 g/L, her other blood tests (white cell count, platelets, electrolytes, calcium and liver function tests) were normal. The Emergency Department doctor diagnosed breathlessness due to anaemia and arranged for her to be admitted for a blood transfusion. The junior doctor on the Acute Medical Unit also assessed the patient and said the same thing. At 11 pm the senior resident doctor reviewed the patient's case and said the same thing. Someone had requested a highly sensitive troponin T in the Emergency Department because the patient had mentioned brief palpitations, although she never had any chest pain. The troponin result was 126 ng/L (normal range 0–13 ng/L). The senior doctor requested a repeat electrocardiogram and troponin test.

*What are your thoughts at this point?*

The next morning another senior resident doctor and an oncology nurse specialist saw the patient and made preparations for a blood transfusion. Then the medical consultant saw the patient. Something did not seem quite right – the patient's haemoglobin was 84 g/L when she did not have symptoms, so

---

*ABC of Clinical Reasoning*, First Edition. Edited by Nicola Cooper and John Frain.

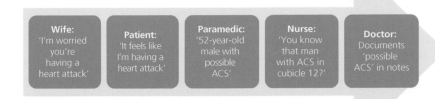

**Figure 5.1** Diagnostic momentum. ACS=acute coronary syndrome.

why was she breathless now? And what was this troponin result all about? It seemed very unlikely she had a heart condition since she never had any chest pain and her 12-lead electrocardiogram was normal. On further questioning, the patient said she was in the supermarket the day before when she suddenly felt light-headed, with associated palpitations and breathlessness. This lasted around 10 minutes and then settled down, but she had 'not felt quite right' since. An urgent computed tomography pulmonary angiogram showed bilateral proximal pulmonary emboli.

Diagnostic momentum (see Figure 5.1) is the tendency for a diagnosis to 'stick' despite lack of supporting evidence. It involves several intermediaries – often starting as an opinion that may not even be medical (e.g. the patient or a relative) – and is passed with increasing certainty from one person to the next. Diagnostic labels become particularly sticky if a specialist has seen the patient.

However, there were several other things going on in this case, for example:

• Anchoring
• Search satisficing
• Confirmation bias
• The effects of night shift work (see Chapter 6)

## Anchoring

Anchoring describes the common human tendency to rely too heavily on the first piece of information offered (the 'anchor') when making decisions. The initial piece of information (in this case, anaemia) is used to make subsequent judgements. Once an anchor is set, other judgements are made by adjusting away from the anchor, and there is a bias towards interpreting other information around it. Businesses use anchoring all the time – the 'recommended retail price' is an anchor. Salespeople use anchors to open negotiations. Several experiments have demonstrated the anchoring effect. In one example, estate agents were asked to estimate the value of a house. Beforehand they were given a randomly generated listed sales price. The higher the listed sales price, the higher they valued the property, although they denied being influenced by the anchor. Lots of studies show that anchoring is very difficult to avoid, although experts may be more resistant to anchoring bias in their particular field.

## Search satisficing

Search satisficing is a term derived from the words 'satisfy' and 'suffice' – when we stop searching because we have found something that fits or is convenient, instead of systematically looking for the best alternative, which involves more effort. Satisficing is beneficial in everyday life – for example, when choosing from an extensive menu at a restaurant, or when there is an unlimited amount of information available and it is necessary to eliminate options and make a decision efficiently. However, in groups satisficing can be detrimental – for example, when people settle for a solution everyone can agree on even though it may not be the best one.

## Confirmation bias

Confirmation bias is the tendency to look for confirming evidence to support a theory rather than looking for disconfirming evidence to refute it, even when the latter is clearly present. Experiments have found repeatedly that people tend to test hypotheses in a one-sided way, by searching for evidence consistent with their current hypothesis. In one example, participants read a profile of a woman that described an equal mix of introvert and extrovert behaviours. Later, they had to recall examples of her introversion and extroversion – one group was told this was to assess the woman for a job as a librarian, while the other group was told it was for a job as an estate agent. There was a significant difference between what the groups recalled, with the 'librarian' group recalling more examples of introversion and the 'sales' group recalling more examples of extroverted behaviour.

## Cognitive miser function

Croskerry writes about the 'cognitive miser' function in clinical decision-making (see 'Further reading/resources'). The brain generally seeks to conserve energy and has an overwhelming tendency to revert to type 1 decision-making, which requires less effort, in some cases becoming 'comfortably numb'. Certain conditions lend themselves to slipping into cognitive miser mode – for example, the workload experienced during a typical night shift for a medical senior resident. However, adopting strategies to conserve thinking effort can lead to problems: failure to do a thorough history and examination, accepting opinions from others at face value and adopting a non-sceptical approach. This mindset leads to diagnostic error.

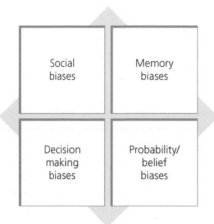

**Figure 5.2** Different types of cognitive biases.

## Common cognitive biases

Cognitive biases are subconscious deviations in judgement leading to perceptual distortion, inaccurate judgement and illogical interpretation. From an evolutionary point of view, they have developed because often speed was more important than accuracy. Biases occur due to information processing shortcuts (or heuristics – see Box 5.1), the brain's limited capacity to process information, social influence, and emotional and moral motivations. The different types of cognitive biases are illustrated in Figure 5.2.

Box 5.2 illustrates some common cognitive biases applicable to healthcare. Biases often work together – for example, in overconfidence bias (the tendency to believe we know more than we actually do) too much faith is placed in opinion instead of gathered evidence. This bias can be augmented by the anchoring effect or availability bias, and finally by commission bias – with disastrous results.

## Is bias only a type 1 thinking problem?

All dual process theories (see Chapter 4) contrast a fast, pattern recognising, intuitive type of thinking, apparently independent of cognitive ability, with a slow, controlled, high effort type of thinking that is strongly associated with cognitive ability and requires access to working memory – see Figure 5.3. In the literature there is an association between type 1 thinking and cognitive biases. While the evidence for dual processing is strong, Evans (see 'Further reading/resources') points out a few problems with

some views of dual process theory. Firstly, it is not true to say that type 1 thinking is responsible for cognitive biases and type 2 thinking is 'the good guy'. There is much evidence that expert decision-making is well served by intuitive rather than analytical/reflective thinking, and sometimes explicit efforts to reason can result in worse performance. People can apply the wrong rules or make errors in their application when it comes to type 2 reasoning. Secondly, while type 1 processing is in general quicker than type 2 processing, it is not true to say that fast processing indicates use of type 1 thinking. Fast type 2 judgements can be made on the basis of simple rules, with minimal reflection. Type 1 judgements can be based on a huge amount of implicit information as is the case with expert intuition.

## Cognitive biases and expert intuition

For many decisions, we lack the necessary information, so we use mental shortcuts and rules of thumb (heuristics). Chapter 7 explores the concept of 'metacognition' – thinking about thinking – and how we might develop strategies to anticipate and reduce errors in our reasoning. However, heuristics are not all bad. Cognitive biases should not be confused with expert intuition, which plays an important role in expert professional practice. The most well-known researcher of expert intuition is Gary Klein (see 'Further reading/resources'). He writes that the more experience people have in any particular field, the more they rely on intuition, which is a natural and direct outgrowth of their *experience* (see Box 5.3 for an example). In this context, he defines intuition as 'the way we translate our experience in to action' – repeated experiences are unconsciously linked together to form patterns. Once we recognise a pattern, we gain sense of a situation, we know what cues to look for and how we should respond. How did the medical consultant *know* the patient in the case history had a pulmonary embolism? It was a combination of recognising risk factors (age, cancer and chemotherapy), linking pulmonary embolism with causes of unexplained breathlessness in past experience, and recognising the blood results did not 'fit' the diagnosis that had been made, but did fit with pulmonary embolism.

Experts bring extensive knowledge and experience to a situation – *but only in their specific domain of expertise*. In 1973, two American psychologists took two groups of people – one consisting of chess masters and one consisting of novices – and showed them chessboards with 20–25 pieces on them, set up as if in the middle of a game. The subjects were shown the boards briefly and then asked to recall the positions of the pieces. The chess masters were able to recall the position of every piece on the board, but the novices could only recall four or five. The experiment was then repeated, but this time the pieces were randomly distributed on the chess board. This time, the chess masters were no better than the novices. Chess masters, with their years of experience, could look at the chess pieces in the middle of a game and see a pattern. The chess pieces were like letters in a word, and like readers recognise whole words, chess masters are experts in the language of chess. But if they were asked to simply look at a jumble of letters, they performed no

Box 5.2 **Common cognitive biases**

**Anchoring**
describes the common human tendency to rely too heavily on the first piece of information offered (the 'anchor') when making decisions.

**Ascertainment Bias**
is when we see what we expect to see ('self-fulfilling prophecy'). For example, a frequent self-harmer attends the ED with drowsiness – everyone assumes he has taken another overdose and misses a brain injury.

**Attribution Error**
is the process of inferring the causes of events or behaviours. For example, if a patient gets better after a certain treatment (y), we might assume the diagnosis must be x.

**Availability Bias**
is when things are at the forefront of your mind because you have seen several cases recently or have been studying that condition in particular. For example, when the author worked in an epilepsy clinic, all blackouts were possible seizures.

**Base Rate Neglect**
is the tendency to ignore the prevalence of a disease which then distorts Bayesian reasoning (see Chapter 3). In some cases, clinicians do this deliberately in order to rule out an unlikely but worse case scenario.

**Commission Bias**
is the tendency towards action rather than inaction, in the assumption that only good can come from doing something (rather than 'watching and waiting').

**Confirmation Bias**
is the tendency to look for confirming evidence to support a theory rather than looking for disconfirming evidence to refute it, even if the latter is clearly present. Confirmation bias is common when a patient has been seen first by another doctor (e.g. GP or ED doctor).

**Diagnostic Momentum**
Once a diagnostic label has been attached to a patient (by the patient or other healthcare professionals) it can gather momentum with each review leading others to exclude other possibilities in their thinking.

**Framing Effect**
is when how a case is presented, for example in handover, can generate bias in the listener. This can be mitigated by always having 'healthy scepticism' about other people's diagnoses.

**Gambler's Fallacy**
is the mistaken belief that if something happens more frequently than normal, then it will happen less frequently in the future (or vice versa). In situations where what is being observed is random, this belief is false.

**Hindsight Bias**
is when knowing the outcome profoundly influences the perception of past events and decision-making, preventing a realistic appraisal of what actually occurred – a major problem in learning from diagnostic error.

**Multiple Alternatives Bias**
is when there are several possibilities, leading to significant uncertainty. This is made easier by reverting to a smaller, more familiar subset of options, which can result in the exclusion of other possibilities.

**Omission Bias**
is the tendency towards inaction, rooted in the principle of 'first do no harm'. Events that occur through natural progression of disease are more acceptable than those that may be attributed directly to the action of the healthcare team.

**Order Effects**
is about the fact that we tend to remember the beginning and the end of information presented to us, not all of it – important to remember in handovers.

**Overconfidence Bias**
is the tendency to believe we know more than we actually do, placing too much faith in opinion instead of gathered evidence.

**Posterior Probability**
occurs when our estimate of the likelihood of disease is unduly influenced by what has gone on before for a particular patient – for example, a patient who has been extensively investigated for headaches presents with a severe headache and serious causes are discounted.

**Premature Closure**
is the tendency to prematurely close the decision-making process and accept a diagnosis before it, and other possibilities, have been fully explored.

**Psych-Out Error**
Psychiatric patients who present with medical problems are under-assessed, under-examined and under-investigated because problems are presumed to be due to, or exacerbated by, their psychiatric condition.

**Representativeness**
'If it looks like a duck, walks like a duck, then it is a duck'. However, this kind of pattern recognising (mistaking 'similar' for 'same') can lead to atypical presentations of diseases being missed.

**Search Satisficing**
is when we stop searching because we have found something that fits or is convenient, instead of systematically looking for the best alternative, which involves more effort.

**Sutton's Slip**
takes its name from a Brooklyn bank robber who explained he robbed banks 'because that's where the money is!' – the strategy of going for the obvious is referred to as Sutton's Law, the slip occurs when other possibilities are not considered.

**Triage-Cueing**
Triage ensures patients get sent to the right department. However, this leads to 'geography is destiny' – for example, a diabetic ketoacidosis patient with abdominal pain and vomiting gets sent to surgery. The wrong location (surgical ward) stops people thinking about medical causes of abdominal pain and vomiting.

**Unpacking Principle**
is when failure to 'unpack' all the available information means things get missed. For example, if a thorough history is not obtained from either the patient or carers (a common problem in Geriatric Medicine) diagnostic possibilities may be discounted.

**Visceral Bias**
refers to the influence of either negative or positive feelings towards patients, which can affect our decision-making.

GP=General Practitioner; ED=Emergency Department.
Adapted from Croskerry P. Achieving quality in clinical decision making: cognitive strategies and detection of bias. *Acad Emerg Med 2002; 9:1184–204.*

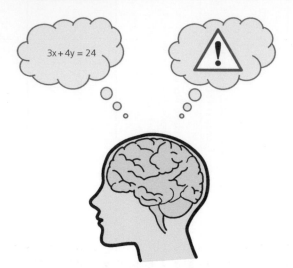

**Figure 5.3** Dual process theory, or the 'two-minds' hypothesis.

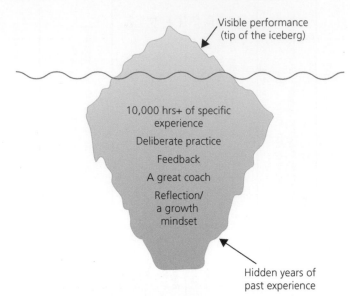

**Figure 5.4** The apparent effortlessness of expert intuition. For example, when you watch a great tennis player you might be forgiven for thinking you are watching effortless talent – what you cannot see is that they started playing tennis aged 4, practised for hours a day for many years, engaged in deliberate practice with the best coaches, and had the determination to learn from mistakes and improve. It is this that underpins the apparent 'effortless' performance, and what we observe in medicine as expert intuition.

---

### Box 5.3 **The neonatal nurse**

Klein tells the story of an experienced neonatal nurse working on an intensive care unit. Towards the end of an uneventful shift the nurse walked past a colleague's patient and noticed 'it didn't look right'. The baby was under the care of a junior colleague who had been monitoring the vital signs all night. The baby had been lethargic, but then babies sleep most of the time. Its temperature had been a little low compared to previously but still within the normal range. A heel prick blood sample had been performed earlier in the shift and the Band Aid on the baby's heel showed it had bled, causing a dark blot. The experienced nurse looked more closely. The baby seemed off colour. She looked at the charts and asked her junior colleague whether the baby seemed more lethargic that shift. When the colleague said yes, the experienced nurse went to the telephone.

The baby had sepsis. The experienced nurse knew this, and organised immediate antibiotics and blood cultures, which were later positive. The signs were *obvious* to her – but not to her junior colleague, who had noted the individual signs but not put them together in a pattern because she had never seen neonatal sepsis before.

---

illogical interpretation. Intelligence and experience do not make a person immune to cognitive biases, and errors can occur in both type 1 and type 2 thinking. However, there is also evidence that expert decision-making can be well served by intuitive thinking. So while healthcare professionals need to be aware of their thinking in order to mitigate the impact of cognitive biases, this does not mean that *intuition in itself* is a bias that needs to be discarded. In fact, expert professional practice can be nurtured by deliberate effort to build a vast databank of experiences that – combined with feedback on our decision-making processes and reflection – allow us in time to recognise patterns, gain sense of a situation, know what to look for and how to respond, while at the same time think about our thinking.

better than everyone else. This 'chunking' of individual pieces into a whole is explained further in Chapter 9.

Expert intuition is really synonymous with tacit knowledge. Although it involves intuitive thinking, this is slightly different to the subconscious 'assumptions' to which we are all prone, experts included, as illustrated in Box 5.2. The apparent effortlessness (which is in fact not effortless at all) of expert intuition is illustrated in Figure 5.4 and has important implications for teaching and learning clinical reasoning.

## Summary

Cognitive biases are everywhere in everyday life and in clinical practice. Cognitive biases are subconscious deviations in judgement leading to perceptual distortion, inaccurate judgement and

## Further reading/resources

Croskerry P. Bias: a normal operating characteristic of the diagnosing brain. *Diagnosis* 2014; **1**:23–7.

Croskerry P. Clinical decision making. In: Barach P, Jacobs L, Lipshultz SE, Laussen P (eds), *Pediatric and Congenital Cardiac Care: Vol. 2: Quality Improvement and Patient Safety*. London: Springer-Verlag, 2015; pp. 397–409.

Dobelli R. *The Art of Thinking Clearly: Better Thinking, Better Decisions*. Sceptre, 2014.

Evans J St BT. Dual process theories of deductive reasoning: facts and fallacies. In: Holyoad KJ and Morrison RG (eds), *The Oxford Handbook of Thinking and Reasoning*. Oxford: Oxford University Press, 2012, pp. 115–33.

Klein G. *The Power of Intuition*. New York: Currency-Doubleday, 2003.

Syed M. Bounce. *The Myth of Talent and the Power of Practice*. London: Fourth Estate, 2011.

## CHAPTER 6

# Human Factors

*Nicola Cooper*

Derby Teaching Hospitals NHS Foundation Trust; and University of Nottingham, UK

---

**OVERVIEW**

- 'Human factors' is the umbrella term used to describe the way people interact with each other, the systems in which they work, and technology

- Human factors covers the design of equipment, systems and processes in order to make it easy for people to do the right thing

- Basic human factors training covers an understanding of error, the limitations of human performance and communication within teams

- Human factors training can improve team performance

- Individuals who understand human factors can act more safely and reduce the chances of error

---

## Introduction

'Human factors' is the umbrella term used to describe the way people interact with each other, the systems in which they work, and technology. The understanding of human factors and how it applies to healthcare has largely derived from the aviation industry as well as other safety critical industries such as nuclear power and the military. Research shows that human factors play a significant role in the majority of accidents. For example, accident analyses, simulator research and cockpit voice recordings show that unsafe flight conditions are frequently related to failures in *cognitive and communication skills* rather than a lack of technical knowledge. Similar contributory causes are found when accidents in the operating theatre are analysed.

In 2013, the Department of Health, along with several other organisations including Health Education England and NHS Employers, signed a human factors in healthcare concordat – stating that:

> The principles and practices of human factors focus on optimising human performance through better understanding the behaviour of individuals, their interactions with each other and with their environment. By acknowledging human limitations, human factors offers ways to minimise

and mitigate human frailties, so reducing medical error and its consequences. The system-wide adoption of these concepts offers a unique opportunity to support cultural change and empower the National Health Service to put patient safety and clinical excellence at its heart.

Human factors is completely integrated into all aspects of aviation education, and pilots are schooled thoroughly in methods of communication. This training is continuous, not a one-off, and it includes everyone. While all pilots have to pass human factors assessments, many healthcare professionals, arguably working in a more unpredictable environment, may never even have heard of the term. In a nutshell, basic human factors training covers:
- An understanding of error
- The limitations of human performance
- Communication within teams

Human factors is also sometimes called 'ergonomics', an established scientific discipline used in many safety critical industries. For the purposes of this chapter, ergonomics – a critical aspect of human factors – is about the design of equipment, workspaces, systems and processes that makes it easy for people to do the right thing. This includes staffing ratios, duty times and rest periods. This chapter will focus more on what might be called 'cognitive ergonomics' – how the limitations of the human brain and poor communication within teams make diagnostic error and other accidents more likely to happen.

What has human factors got to do with clinical reasoning? Chapter 5 explored the common cognitive biases that occur in everyday life as well as in clinical practice. Human factors includes cognitive biases as well as 'affective biases' (how cognition is affected by our emotions and the environment) with an emphasis on clinical teams and the workplace.

## Error in healthcare

Until 1991, there was little information on the scale of adverse events within healthcare. See Box 6.1 for some definitions. We now know from a multitude of studies that healthcare can be

---

unsafe – one UK study showed that adverse events occurred in around 10% of hospital admissions, directly leading to death in 1% of cases. Around half of the adverse events were judged to be preventable. In 2014 there were 15 million hospital admissions in the UK.

Research shows that *errors are predictable and tend to repeat themselves in patterns*. Healthcare staff do not come to work to deliberately harm patients, rather 'to err is human'. We, the systems in which we work, and the processes that are in place, can either adapt for this and make error and adverse events less likely, or can in fact create 'accidents waiting to happen'. This is what human factors is all about.

Figure 6.1 shows an everyday example of human factors engineering. Healthcare equipment is often not designed with human cognitive limitations in mind. Poor design is a frequent cause of patient safety incidents. When healthcare organisations use a large number of different medical devices there is an increased risk that staff will make errors. The National Patient Safety Agency found that, on average, UK hospitals had 31 different types of infusion devices in use and there was no clinical reason for this diversity. It has issued a safety notice recommending that healthcare organisations minimise the number of different medical devices in use.

Serious adverse events tend to occur after a series of smaller things go wrong – this is referred to as an 'error chain', illustrated by the Swiss cheese model of accident causation described by James Reason (see Figure 6.2).

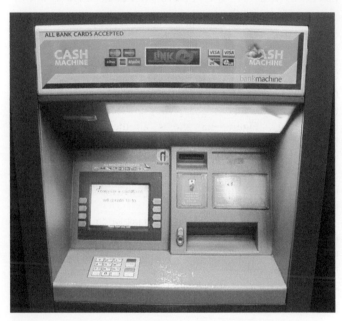

**Figure 6.1** Everyday example of human factors engineering – a cash machine, or ATM. Cash machines around the world have the same design – from the arrangement of the numbers on the keypad to the fact that the machine beeps and flashes to remind you to take your card *before* it dispenses your cash. This is an example of human factors engineering, design that takes into account that 'to err is human'. How many of us would walk off leaving our cards behind if cashpoint machines did not operate this way?

---

Box 6.1 **Definitions**

- An 'adverse event' is an unintended injury caused by the healthcare system rather than the disease process itself.
- An adverse event may or may not be preventable – for example, a patient with anaphylaxis to penicillin may have had no known allergies, therefore the adverse event could not have been prevented. It is estimated that around half of adverse events are preventable.
- The number of clinical errors is far higher than the number of adverse events – this is because errors may not cause harm or they may be intercepted in time (e.g. an incorrect prescription).
- For every major adverse event, there are around 29 minor injuries and 300 'no harm accidents' (known as the Heinrich ratio) – adverse events are the tip of the iceberg. This is important because we can learn far more about *why* things go wrong by analysing the greater number of minor incidents that occur, which is why incident reporting is mandatory and confidential in the aviation industry.

---

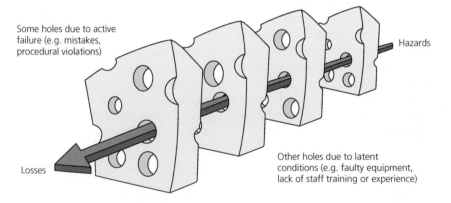

**Figure 6.2** Swiss cheese model of accident causation. For example, blood transfusion has a series of defences, barriers and safeguards, from donation to screening to storage to administration. But in any human system, these defences can have holes in them – like Swiss cheese. If the conditions are wrong and these holes happen to align, a major adverse event can occur. The important thing to understand is that in order to prevent an adverse event from happening again, the latent conditions – or 'root causes' – must be addressed. Errors rarely happen because of the actions of one person. Reproduced with permission from Reason, J. *Human Error*. Cambridge University Press, 1990.

Simplified processes, standardised ways of doing things, equipment design, thorough induction and training, electronic prescribing – these are a few examples of ways in which healthcare can mitigate the 'human factor'. However, individuals also need to understand how the human brain is wired and how they can act in a way that makes errors and adverse events less likely.

## The limitations of human performance

Humans are not perfect. The human brain is wired to miss things that are obvious, see patterns that do not exist, and jump to conclusions. Take a look at Box 6.2, but only for a few moments, enough to read the sentence twice. How many 'F's are there?

When this experiment is given to a room full of people, there is a range of opinion. Some people see two 'F's, some see three, some see four, five or six. This is a group of highly intelligent people (usually doctors) who can all read English, who are all looking at the same thing – yet as a group they are seeing differently from one another. Figure 6.3 shows another simple example. Experiments like these are used to teach something called 'situation awareness'. Individuals can have situation awareness and see what is going on, but a team's situation awareness can be low if no one communicates, especially when something appears to be obvious (see Box 6.3).

Drew and colleagues from Harvard asked 23 consultant radiologists to look at CT scans of the thorax specifically to look for lung nodules. Unknown to the radiologists, the researchers inserted a matchbox-sized image of a gorilla in some of the scans. They found that 83% of the radiologists missed the gorilla, which was 45 times larger than the average lung nodule, even though they spent an average of 5.7 seconds looking at the gorilla-containing images and their eyes fixed briefly on the exact location of the gorilla.

This experiment highlights that we are only aware of a small part of our visual world at any one time. We focus our attention to filter out distractions, but in focusing on what we are trying to see, we tend not to notice the unexpected. This explains why in the past, many patients were killed by accidental injections of potassium chloride solution, which was stored alongside sodium chloride (used as a flush) in identical packaging on wards. A human *expecting to see* sodium chloride could easily read the label yet miss that it said potassium chloride. The answer to this problem was straightforward – potassium chloride is no longer stocked on wards.

Humans also see patterns that do not exist and have a tendency to 'fill in the gaps', make assumptions and jump to conclusions. Daniel Kahneman's book, *Thinking, Fast and Slow* (Allen Lane, London, 2011) sets out the broad theme that human beings are intuitive thinkers and that human intuition is imperfect. Box 6.4 shows one of his examples.

As James Reason said, 'Good doctors are *not* those who don't make mistakes; good doctors are those who expect to make mistakes and act on that expectation.'

Our perceptions and performance can be fallible at the best of times, but are also adversely affected by:
- Night work
- Fatigue
- Stress
- Excessive workload/cognitive overload
- Illness

---

Box 6.2 **How many 'F's are there?**

Take only a few moments to read the following sentence twice:

> FINISHED FILES ARE THE RESULTS OF
> YEARS OF SCIENTIFIC STUDY
> COMBINED WITH THE EXPERIENCE
> OF YEARS

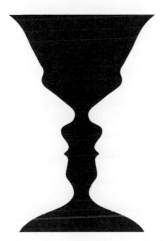

**Figure 6.3** Optical illusions. Do you see the vase or the faces?

---

Box 6.3 **Situation awareness**

'A light aircraft is heading towards an airport surrounded by mountains. The captain has inadvertently descended below the minimum safe altitude and the aircraft is on a collision course with the mountain. It is the co-pilot's first day and he can see that the aircraft is headed towards the mountain. The captain is experienced and has flown this route many times before. He is bored and preoccupied with problems at home. The co-pilot reasons that such an experienced captain surely knows what he is doing. Is there any need to say anything?'

From McAllister B. *Crew Resource Management. Awareness, Cockpit Efficiency and Safety.* Shrewsbury: Airlife Publishing Ltd, 1997.

---

Box 6.4 **The lazy system 1**

Here is a simple puzzle. Do not try to solve it but listen to your intuition:

> A bat and ball cost $1.10
> The bat costs one dollar more than the ball.
> How much does the ball cost?

A number came to your mind – 10c. Most people come up with this answer. As Kahneman says, it is intuitive, appealing, and *wrong* (the correct answer is 5c).

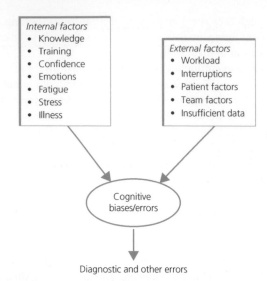

**Figure 6.4** Factors increasing the likelihood of diagnostic error.

In one survey, 75% of pilots said that fatigue affected their performance, but only 30% of surgeons said the same. In fact, research shows that lack of sleep impacts on performance significantly. Registrars in obstetrics and gynaecology participated in one experiment (D. Dawson and K. Reid. Fatigue, alcohol and performance impairment. *Nature* 1997: 388;235) in which one group worked a 24-hour shift and the other group (not at work) was given alcohol. Cognitive psychometric testing was performed at regular intervals. After 17 hours of sustained wakefulness (3 am) performance decreased to a level equivalent to a blood alcohol concentration of 0.05% – the driving limit in most Western countries. At the end of the shift (8 am) performance was equivalent to a blood alcohol concentration of 0.1% – the reason 24-hour shifts no longer exist in the UK.

Chapter 4 described dual process theory – type 1 and type 2 thinking. The pathways in the brain involved in type 2 processing (the deliberate, analytical type of thinking) are most affected by things like sleep deprivation, fatigue and cognitive overload. Figure 6.4 shows how lots of factors combine to increase the likelihood of cognitive biases, resulting in diagnostic and other errors.

How can an individual mitigate against the limitations of human performance? The following tips are taken from the 'how to guide' for implementing human factors in healthcare (see 'Further reading/resources'):

• Be self-aware. If you are stressed and having trouble concentrating, consider yourself at greater risk of making a mistake and act accordingly.
• In emergency situations quickly allocate a leader. Rehearse emergency drills as a team.
• Perform complex drug calculations away from distractions and get them checked by someone else.
• Don't rely on your memory. The human brain can only have seven or eight things at its forefront at any one time. Use checklists and standard operating procedures to improve compliance with best practice.

---

Box 6.5 **Training courses in human factors (non-technical skills)**

In the UK, the postgraduate courses such as Anaesthetists' Non-Technical Skills (ANTS) have been developed. They focus on cognitive (awareness, decision-making) and interpersonal skills. This training improves the performance of clinical teams.

The domains of ANTS training:

| Teamwork | Task management |
| --- | --- |
| Co-ordinating activities with the team | Planning and preparing |
| Exchanging information | Prioritising |
| Using authority and assertiveness | Providing and maintaining standards |
| Assessing capabilities | Identifying and utilising |
| Supporting others | resources |
| *Situation awareness* | *Decision-making* |
| Gathering information | Identifying options |
| Recognising and understanding | Balancing risks and selecting options |
| Anticipating | Re-evaluating |

• ANTS: Anaesthetists' Non-Technical Skills System Handbook. University of Aberdeen and Scottish Clinical Simulation Centre, 2001. Available from: http://www.abdn.ac.uk/iprc/documents/ants/ants_handbook_v1.0_electronic_access_version.pdf (accessed February 2016).
• NOTSS: Non-Technical Skills for Surgeons System Handbook v 1.2. 2006. University of Aberdeen. Available from: www.abdn.ac.uk/iprc/notss (accessed 18 February 2016).
• SPLINTS: Scrub Practitioners' List of Intraoperative Non-Technical Skills Handbook. University of Aberdeen, 2009. Available from: www.abdn.ac.uk/iprc/splints (accessed 18 February 2015).

• Be aware that humans often see what they expect to see – this is known as 'involuntary automaticity'.
• If a task requires focus and concentration, ensure you cannot be distracted.
• Simplify your environment and clinical processes as far as possible.

## Communication within teams

Communication within teams is extremely important when flawed human beings are working in flawed systems and busy clinical environments full of interruptions. Specific training courses exist in the UK for human factors or 'non-technical skills', and form part of postgraduate training programmes for theatre teams (see Box 6.5 for details).

For effective communication to occur, the message needs to be clear in the first place. Then the message has to get through competing demands to the recipient. Then it has to be heard, interpreted and translated into action. The majority of adverse events include failure in communication as a root cause.

Clear communication involves:
• Stating the obvious
• Announcing what you are doing
• *Not* using pronouns (e.g. he, she, it, they)

- Using 'readback' – repeating back information to ensure it is correct
- Clearly stating what you want from someone
- Clearly articulating safety concerns
- Listening to others

For example, as a junior doctor, the author was on a respiratory ward round. The consultant, registrar, author and ward sister were all looking at a chest X-ray. After several minutes, the doctors declared it was normal – until the ward sister pointed out the huge pneumothorax on the left side. She almost did not speak up, thinking the abnormality was so *obvious*. But in several cases of wrong site surgery in the UK, there was someone in theatre who knew it was the wrong side, but did not feel able to speak up. The World Health Organization's safe surgery checklist, includes a 'time out' before each operation, during which team members must confirm the identity of the patient and the correct site (including side) of the procedure.

Announcing what you are doing is vital in emergency situations where an entire team is working simultaneously – it would be very easy to accidentally administer the same drug again, or not give it at all thinking that someone else has already done it. 'Problematic pronouns' are rife in clinical practice. In hospitals, staff members frequently refer to he/she/it/they instead of the patient's name and location – without realising how easily this can lead to errors. The use of 'readback' for verbal orders (e.g. for medication) and messages (e.g. telephoned blood results) also significantly reduces error.

The SBAR (situation, background, assessment, recommendation) system of communication originated in the military and is illustrated in Box 6.6. In healthcare, it has been shown to increase the amount of relevant information being communicated and in a shorter time. Probably the most useful component of SBAR is the final part – recommendation – in which the messenger clearly states what they would like to happen next. Think about how many times someone has simply told you a story without actually stating what they would like you to do.

Finally, clearly articulating safety concerns and listening to others is vital, as in the scenario in Box 6.3. Other people may simply not see what you can see, no matter how experienced they are – *to err is human*. 'Red flags' are warnings – often occurring in the minutes leading up to an adverse event. Examples of red flags are shown in Box 6.7. A red flag is a cue for action. It means you have to stop to communicate with the rest of the team so the situation can be reassessed.

## Embedding human factors in healthcare

How does healthcare adopt human factors – from an overall understanding of error to design of equipment, workspaces, rotas, systems and processes that make it easy for people to do the right thing; the limitations of human performance and communication within teams?

One way is to introduce human factors training – for everyone. Fire safety training, for example, is mandatory for staff in healthcare

---

**Box 6.6 The SBAR system of communicating**

**S   Situation**
I am [name/designation] calling from [location]
The reason I am calling is because I have a patient with a National Early Warning Score of 9 and he needs to be reviewed by a doctor a.s.a.p.

**B   Background**
Patient [name] was admitted on [date] with pneumonia
He is normally fit and well
His oxygen requirements have been increasing throughout the course of the day

**A   Assessment**
His vital signs are [read out vital signs]
I think the problem is…
OR I am not sure what the problem is but [name] is deteriorating
I have [actions performed so far]

**R   Recommendation**
I need you to come and see [name] within the next 30 minutes

The listener can readback a summary of the SBAR. The caller can readback any instructions to ensure that they have been heard correctly.

**Resources**
Patient Safety First: http://www.institute.nhs.uk/safer_care/general/patient_safety_first.html (accessed February 2016).
National Early Warning Score (NEWS). Standardising the assessment of acute illness severity in the NHS. Royal College of Physicians of London, 2012. Available at: https://www.rcplondon.ac.uk/resources/national-early-warning-score-news (accessed February 2016)

---

**Box 6.7 Red flags**

A red flag, or warning, often occurs in the minutes leading up to an adverse event. Examples of red flags include:

- Confusion
- Conflicting or missing information
- Departure from standard procedure
- Unease
- Denial or irritability
- Inaction
- Alarms
- Alarming thoughts

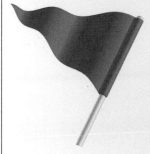

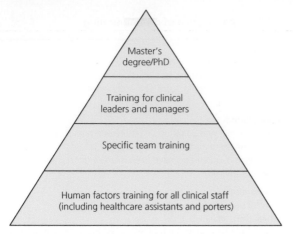

**Figure 6.5** A human factors training 'hierarchy'. A human factors training programme in healthcare must include basic training for all staff, adapted to suit their roles. Specific team training (e.g. theatres, delivery suite, emergency department) is also important. Clinical leaders and managers need a greater awareness of system, process and equipment design. Some people can gain a master's degree or even PhD in Ergonomics and Human Factors and become a project leader and mentor in an organisation.

organisations in the UK, yet adverse events in healthcare, in which human factors play a large part, harm far more people than fire. Figure 6.5 illustrates a human factors training 'hierarchy' that could be implemented in a typical healthcare organisation.

## Summary

Expertise, competence and hard work do not on their own safeguard against errors that result in harm. Healthcare staff who are trained to understand 'to err is human' can ensure their workplace and processes are designed with human factors in mind, and ensure they act in ways that are safe – including understanding the effect of fatigue and stress on performance and communicating with other team members in a way that enhances patient safety.

## Further reading/resources

Clinical Human Factors Group. Website: www.chfg.org (accessed 18 February 2016).

Gawande A. *The Checklist Manifesto: How to Get Things Right*. Profile Books, 2011.

Gordon S, Mendenhall P, O'Connor BB. *Beyond the Checklist: What Else Healthcare can Learn from Aviation Teamwork and Safety*. ILR Press, 2012.

Human factors in healthcare. A concordat from the National Quality Board. London, 2013. Available at: https://www.england.nhs.uk/wp-content/uploads/2013/11/nqb-hum-fact-concord.pdf (accessed 18 February 2016).

The 'How to Guide' for Implementing Human Factors in Healthcare. Patient Safety First Campaign. Available at: http://www.chfg.org/resources/10_qrt01/Human_Factors_How_to_Guide_2009.pdf (accessed 18 February 2016).

Vincent C, Neale G, Woloshynowych M. Adverse events in British Hospitals: preliminary retrospective record review. *BMJ* 2001; **322**:517–19.

# CHAPTER 7

# Metacognition and Cognitive Debiasing

*Pat Croskerry*

Dalhousie University, Halifax, Nova Scotia, Canada

---

### OVERVIEW

- Metacognition is 'thinking about thinking'
- Metacognition can be used to reduce the impact of biases and improve clinical decision-making
- Some established clinical practices have built in debiasing strategies
- Developing 'mindware' for specific biases can also improve clinical decision-making
- Cognitive debiasing is not easy – it requires multiple strategies, multiple efforts and lifelong maintenance

---

## Introduction

Imagine that you are walking out of a morbidity and mortality meeting in your hospital in which two cases of diagnostic failure have just been discussed. Your colleagues are chatting about the cases. The first involved a 17-year-old whose diagnosis of meningitis was delayed, and the second was a 66-year-old whose acute myocardial infarction was missed. A detailed discussion led to the conclusion that cognitive errors were involved in both cases. In the first, the main error was identified as confirmation bias in that the physician appeared to avoid doing a lumbar puncture, confirming to himself instead that the patient's symptoms of fever, headache, and neck 'spasms' were consistent with a flu-like illness. In the second, the errors were identified as framing and search satisficing in a woman who had developed shoulder pain while mowing her lawn, and was diagnosed with a shoulder sprain. One of your colleagues appears knowledgeable about cognitive errors and suggests they might have been avoided and diagnostic failure averted if the physicians involved had been more familiar with cognitive biases and how to deal with them. You wonder out loud why you did not hear more about cognitive biases and debiasing while you were in medical school.

It is now widely accepted that there are two principal modes of decision-making, referred to as dual process theory: fast, intuitive type 1 thinking, and slow, analytical type 2 thinking (discussed in more detail in Chapter 4). If type 1 thinking is faster, why do we not use it all the time, instead of deferring to the slower type 2, especially in situations that have time and cost restraints? The answer is that while type 1 thinking works well most of the time, it does not work well *all* of the time. Taking shortcuts and using abbreviated ways of thinking (heuristics) often involves biases, and placing our faith in type 1 thinking may lead to costly errors.

Nevertheless, we spend most of our time in type 1 mode and people generally prefer being there. It is the constant default state of the conscious mind and requires considerably less effort than type 2 thinking. If, as it strongly appears, bias will inevitably enter our decision-making, perhaps the most appropriate approach to improving decision-making is to adopt strategies to overcome the negative aspects of biases. This strategy requires *metacognition*, the ability to pull back from the immediate situation and think about the thinking underlying our decision-making – the focus of this chapter.

## 'Brutish automatism'

We spend our conscious time in either a passive or an active state. Passive consciousness is adequate for most of what we do. You can observe it for yourself in everyday life, for example driving a car. Most of the time we spend driving is passive. We execute the complex psychological, motor, and haptic (sense of touch) tasks necessary to keep the car moving in a safe and effective manner, and do enough to get by. This is a default state rather than a deliberate choice.

However, you can deliberately change your driving to an active state. Look down and check the instruments: is there anything abnormal? Am I in the correct gear? Is my speed appropriate for the limit and the conditions? Am I too close to the car in front? Would I have enough time to react if a tyre suddenly blew or a child ran into the road? This active state requires vigilance that typically challenges the status quo by asking questions and making predictions about the future.

---

*ABC of Clinical Reasoning*, First Edition. Edited by Nicola Cooper and John Frain.

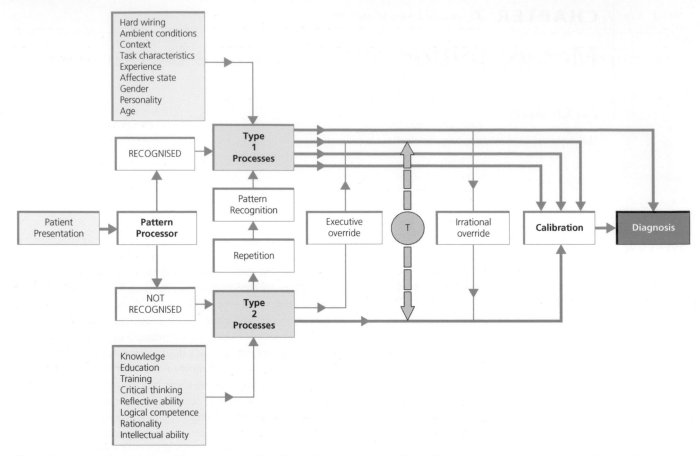

**Figure 7.1** A schematic application of dual process model to diagnostic decision-making. The multi-channelled type 1 processes depict fast, intuitive decision-making, and the single-channelled type 2 process analytical decision-making. The executive override pathway shows type 2 surveillance and potential override of type 1 decision-making and provides the means for accomplishing metacognition and cognitive debiasing. The lower shaded box contains the mindware for debiasing.

Being able to monitor one's thinking and distinguishing between the two states is important. In a broader context of awareness, Durrell saw it as our biggest challenge: 'The greatest delicacy of judgement, the greatest refinement of intention was to replace the brutish automatism with which most of us exist, stuck like prehistoric animals in the sludge of our non-awareness'. (Lawrence Durrell, *A Smile in the Mind's Eye: An Adventure into Zen Philosophy*. Open Road Media, London, 2012).

Replacing Durrell's 'brutish automatism' and unsticking ourselves from the 'sludge of non-awareness' requires the active process of metacognition – a key concept in clinical reasoning. It is thinking about what we are currently thinking in the immediate environment, and also of the role that we are playing in the immediate process. Above all, metacognition is the pathway towards developing improvement strategies in our decision-making, and dual process theory gives us the scaffold for the job. When type 2 thinking is used to actively monitor the decisions being made in type 1 mode we are said to be engaging metacognition. This active surveillance of type 1 thinking is the first step in developing good reasoning skills. It is also referred to as 'executive override', as Figure 7.1 illustrates.

## Cognitive debiasing

### Established strategies

Although the experimental evidence for cognitive biases has emerged only in the last 40 years, clinicians have long been aware of the intrusion of bias into clinical reasoning. Historically, a number of strategies were developed to deal with biases, faulty reasoning and memory deficits (see Table 7.1). They were regarded as self-evident and have not been subjected to formal experimental validation.

Taking a history and performing a physical examination were established in modern medicine to gather data in a systematic way so that important information was not missed. Systematic history taking and physical examination were both strategies developed to support the *unpacking principle* – the more information gleaned, the greater likelihood of not missing something important. Despite the proven usefulness of gathering such data, there are still those prepared to make *Augenblick* (blink of an eye) or 'spot' diagnoses, often in the context of a 'corridor consultation'. 'Spot diagnoses', said the eminent surgeon Sir Zachary Cope, 'were magnificent and impressive, but unsafe'.

**Table 7.1** Established strategies in medicine to mitigate cognitive and affective biases.

| Strategy | Purpose | Examples of biases |
| --- | --- | --- |
| History and physical exam | Systematic gathering of data | 'Augenblick' or spot diagnoses<br>Unpacking principle<br>Ascertainment bias |
| Differential diagnosis | Forces consideration of diagnostic possibilities other than the obvious or the most likely | Anchoring and adjustment<br>Search satisficing<br>Premature diagnostic closure<br>Availability bias<br>Representativeness<br>Confirmation bias |
| Clinical prediction rules | Force a scientific, statistical assessment of the patient's symptoms, signs and other data to develop numerical probabilities of the presence/absence of a disease or an outcome | Base rate fallacy<br>Errors of reasoning |
| Evidence-based medicine | Establishes imperative for objective scientific data to support analytic decision-making | Biases that arise out of unexamined type 1 decision-making |
| Checklists | Ensure that important issues have been considered and completed, especially under conditions of complexity, stress and fatigue, but also when routine processes are being followed | Anchoring and adjustment<br>Availability bias<br>Memory failures |
| Mnemonics | Protect against memory failures and ensure a full range of possibilities is considered in the differential diagnosis.<br>Forces thinking outside the obvious possibilities | Availability bias<br>Anchoring and adjustment |
| Pitfalls | Alert inexperienced clinicians to predictable failures commonly encountered in a particular discipline | Biases that predictably arise in specific clinical situations |
| ROWS | Ensures that the most serious condition in a particular clinical setting is not missed | Anchoring and adjustment<br>Premature diagnostic closure<br>Search satisficing |
| Caveats | Often discipline-specific warnings to ensure important rules are followed to avoid missing significant conditions | Predictable biases known to specific disciplines |
| Red flags | Specific signs and symptoms to look out for, often in the context of commonly presenting conditions, to avoid missing serious conditions | Framing<br>Search satisficing<br>Premature closure |

The development of the concept of a differential diagnosis in the late nineteenth century by the German psychiatrist Emil Kraepelin was intended to bring order to the classification of psychiatric illnesses, but ultimately enjoyed broader application in medicine by judging the relative likelihood of a particular disease in patients suffering symptoms that might be common to several diseases. Establishing a differential diagnosis implicitly works against *anchoring* onto a particular diagnosis too early in the diagnostic process, thereby avoiding *search satisficing* and perhaps *premature diagnostic closure*. It has a built-in forcing function that requires asking the important question: 'What else could this be?' Electronic applications that provide extensive differential diagnostic checklists are now available.

Although evidence-based medicine is now accepted as a standard of practice, it took a surprisingly long time to emerge. Prior to its acceptance, many clinical practices were pursued and sustained in the absence of any proof of their efficacy. This allowed myths, idiosyncratic beliefs, and often harmful practices to flourish without being challenged. Further, evidence-based medicine brought with it the imperative to critically appraise the evidence to detect biases in the methods used to obtain such evidence.

The use of checklists is long-standing in medicine. The simple ABC (airway-breathing-circulation) in resuscitation provides a forcing function that ensures critical issues are addressed, often under conditions of increased stress. But checklists are also highly effective in ensuring that evidence-based aspects of care (bundles)

Box 7.1 **APGAR Score**

In 1952 Virginia Apgar, an anaesthetist at Columbia University, New York, proposed the first standardised scoring method for evaluating newborn children. A decade later, her surname was used in the mnemonic the APGAR Score, which predicts survival and neurological development.

A – appearance
P – pulse
G – grimace
A – activity
R – respiration

are followed in routine procedures, for example prevention of catheter-related bloodstream infections in the intensive care unit.

Given certain symptoms, signs and other data, clinical prediction rules aim to attach a numeric probability of the likelihood of a specific disorder or outcome. Examples are the Wells' criteria for pulmonary embolus and the Ottawa ankle rules.

Another important adjunct in the clinical armamentarium is mnemonics. Mnemonics are abundant in medicine and serve several important functions. Their major purpose is to reduce reliance on fallible memory, especially of things that are not coherently connected. A classic example is the APGAR score (see Box 7.1), which is both a mnemonic and also a forcing function to assess five critical parameters in the newborn. It has proved to be a valid predictor of neonatal mortality. Another, for causes of high anion gap metabolic acidosis, is 'MUDPILES' (see Box 7.2), which provides a checklist and a forcing function to ensure that a number of unrelated possibilities are considered. More recent applications of mnemonics have proven efficacy, such as a mnemonic-based method for handovers: 'I-PASS' (I – illness severity; P – patient summary; A – action list; S – situation awareness and contingency planning; S – synthesis by receiver).

Most disciplines in medicine identify specific pitfalls to warn inexperienced trainees about clinical situations in which predictable errors commonly occur: for example, 'Always examine the joint above and below the apparent injury in children'. These have emerged over the years and are often spread by word of mouth. Similarly, general and specific caveats have been established in many disciplines; for example, 'Beware the patient who returns to the emergency department', and 'The most commonly missed fracture is the second one'.

The heuristic that rules out the worst case scenario (ROWS) is a forcing function that commits the clinician always to consider the worst possible illness that might explain a particular presentation and take steps to ensure it has been effectively excluded; for example, always consider pulmonary embolus with any patient with chest symptoms or tachycardia, and always consider a scaphoid fracture with a wrist sprain.

Finally, red flags are another form of forcing function that alert clinicians to the possibility of a serious illness that may appear in the context of a common presentation. For example, lower back pain is nearly always what it appears to be: a musculoskeletal problem. But occasionally it is the harbinger of something very serious such as a spinal abscess (red flags: fever plus track marks or a history of intravenous drug use), or cauda equina syndrome (red flags: proximal leg weakness, urinary retention, decreased sphincter tone).

### Newly evolving strategies

Over the last 40 years a number of studies in the behavioural sciences have demonstrated the extensive impact of bias on human judgement and decision-making, and numerous books have appeared on the topic. Fairly early on, notably in the work by Fischoff, efforts were made to develop debiasing strategies. His conclusion, and one that a number of other researchers have since reached, was that debiasing is not easy. This should not be surprising – many biases in decision-making exist either because

they have been selected in an evolutionary sense or have been established through multiple repetitions. They are the status quo of normal brain functioning and are not going to be displaced very easily. Biases by their nature are robust and difficult to change – they would not be biases if they weren't. Nevertheless, there is a prolific interest in developing debiasing strategies, not just in medicine but in all realms of human behaviour. Graber et al. conducted a narrative review that found 42 tested interventions to mitigate diagnostic error, and Croskerry et al. reviewed the theory and practice of debiasing, describing a number of educational and workplace strategies as well as specific forcing functions to accomplish it (see 'Further reading/resources').

Forcing functions are a particularly effective means of changing behaviour. They are anything that forces a particular direction in a response, and can be graded along a spectrum in terms of how rigidly they do so. Nudging strategies simply make it easier for a person to make a desirable response; for example, instead of having one box at the bottom of an emergency chart for the diagnosis, a second box could be provided to allow an NYD (not yet diagnosed) option. This might lessen the tendency to prematurely close on a particular diagnosis if there is still significant uncertainty. More explicit forcing functions can effectively eliminate the possibility of overlooking a significant condition, for example requiring that vital signs are measured in every patient in the emergency department.

### Situational vulnerability to bias

Another approach is to identify specific clinical situations or conditions that might be vulnerable to particular biases (see Table 7.2). Predictable biases are more likely in certain situations, and it is a useful exercise to consider specific biases that may be at play. It is also important to remember that certain conditions (fatigue, sleep deprivation, cognitive overload) increase the proportion of time spent in type 1 mode, as outlined in Chapter 6, and therefore increase the likelihood of bias in decision-making.

### Overall challenges of debiasing

The basic elements of cognitive debiasing are schematised in Figure 7.2. Initially the decision-maker needs to be fully aware of the impact of bias on decision-making. Not everyone is. Some decision-makers may themselves suffer from the metabias *blind-spot bias*, which itself reflects an overall deficiency in reasoning and judgement about cognitive and affective biases. Those with blind-spot bias may deny the importance or impact of biases altogether. Secondly, the decision-maker should be aware of the nature of biases and how they may affect many aspects of brain function, as well as their extent. Despite having this awareness, some may feel that biases are inevitable and difficult to change, and so are not willing to make the effort. This itself is referred to as the *status quo bias*, which some see as a lack of motivation to make the cognitive effort to change. The next step of the process is learning about the specific mindware necessary to effect debiasing.

The important concept of *mindware* was originally developed in 1995 by the Harvard cognitive scientist Perkins to describe the rules, knowledge, procedures and strategies that a decision-maker can retrieve from memory to facilitate sound reasoning and decision-making. Robust mindware provides the decision-maker with the necessary tools to recognise and deal with bias (e.g. knowledge about biases, rationality, scientific thinking, logic) and can extend to specific strategies to deal with particular biases. For example, the mindware to deal with confirmation bias is the knowledge that it can be effectively overcome by looking for and applying disconfirming evidence. The final step of the debiasing process is to implement the appropriate mindware to execute debiasing when the situation calls for it (Figure 7.3). It is also very important that the good habits of debiasing be maintained throughout one's clinical career as older clinicians spend increasing amounts of time using type 1 thinking.

Overall, cognitive debiasing strategies are difficult to implement (see Box 7.3). It is unlikely that one debiasing strategy will work for all, equally unlikely that one shot will be effective, and very likely that maintenance of debiasing will be a necessary part of clinical practice.

**Table 7.2** Examples of biases that are common in certain situations.

| Clinical situation | Examples of potential biases |
| --- | --- |
| Have I reached this diagnosis very quickly? | Overconfidence<br>Anchoring<br>Search satisficing<br>Premature diagnostic closure<br>Unpacking principle |
| Was this patient transferred from another individual/team to me? | Ascertainment bias<br>Framing<br>Diagnostic momentum<br>Premature diagnostic closure |
| Has a diagnosis been suggested to me by the patient, paramedic, nurse or physician? | Anchoring<br>Ascertainment bias<br>Framing<br>Search satisficing<br>Confirmation bias |
| Did I just accept the first diagnosis that came to mind? | Availability<br>Representativeness<br>Search satisficing<br>Premature diagnostic closure |
| Did I consider organ systems other than the obvious one? | Anchoring<br>Search satisficing<br>Premature diagnostic closure |
| Do I dislike this patient, or do they remind me of another patient I don't like? | Visceral bias<br>Availability<br>Fundamental attribution error |
| Am I stereotyping this patient, or do they belong to a group of patients that I may feel negatively about? Have I been fair to the patient? | Representativeness bias<br>Visceral bias<br>Anchoring<br>Fundamental attribution error<br>Availability |
| Was I interrupted or significantly distracted while assessing this patient? | All biases |
| Am I suffering from sleep deprivation right now? | All biases |
| Am I in a hurry, cognitively overloaded, fatigued, or over-extended right now? | All biases |
| Have I effectively ruled out a must-not-miss diagnosis? | Overconfidence<br>Anchoring<br>Search satisficing<br>Confirmation bias |

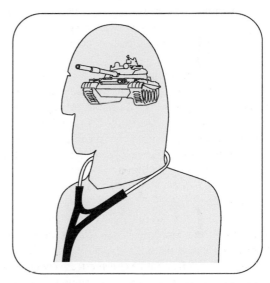

**Figure 7.3** Robust mindware is needed to deal with the wide variety of biases that enter into clinical decision-making.

Box 7.3 **Characteristics of the debiasing process**

- Needs comprehensive knowledge of nature and extent of biases
- Requires development of good mindware
- Generally difficult
- One debiasing strategy will not work for all biases
- One shot unlikely to be effective
- Requires lifelong maintenance

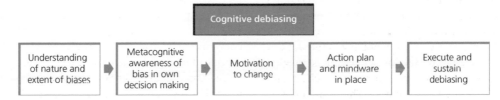

**Figure 7.2** Metacognitive schema for cognitive and affective debiasing.

## Summary

Sound decision-making is one of the most important characteristics of the well-calibrated clinician. While a number of aspects of the clinical decision-making process are important, principal among them is the ability to detect and recognise cognitive and affective biases. This involves metacognition – the process of thinking about thinking.

Historically, medicine has evolved a number of different strategies to mitigate and avoid bias. However, since the unmasking of the nature and extent of cognitive and affective biases over the last four decades, these debiasing strategies can now be further strengthened by developing explicit mindware deliberately aimed at reducing the overall effects of bias on clinical decision making.

## Further reading/resources

Croskerry P, Singhal G, Mamede S. Cognitive debiasing 1: origins of bias and theory of debiasing. *BMJ Qual Saf* 2013; **22**(Suppl 2):ii58–ii64.

Croskerry P, Singhal G, Mamede S. Cognitive debiasing 2: impediments to and strategies for change. *BMJ Qual Saf* 2013; **22**(Suppl 2):ii65–ii72.

Croskerry P. Bias: a normal operating characteristic of the diagnosing brain. *Diagnosis* 2014; **1**:23–7.

Eta S, Berner ES, Graber ML. Overconfidence as a cause of diagnostic error in medicine. *Am J Med* 2008; **121**(5A):S2–S23.

Graber ML, Kissam S, Payne VL et al. Cognitive interventions to reduce diagnostic error: a narrative review. *BMJ Qual Saf* 2012; **21**:535–57.

Milkman KL, Chugh D, Bazerman MH. How can decision making be improved? *Perspect Psychol Sci* 2009; **4**:379–83.

## CHAPTER 8

# Using Guidelines, Scores and Decision Aids

*Maggie Bartlett and Simon Gay*

Keele School of Medicine, Staffordshire, UK

> **OVERVIEW**
> - Clinical reasoning does not stop with a diagnosis
> - Clinical reasoning is needed for subsequent decisions about investigation, management and treatment
> - Using guidelines and other decision aids can help clinicians and patients to make decisions
> - There are some pitfalls involved in using decision aids
> - Patients' values and concerns must be incorporated into the decision-making process

## Introduction

In this chapter, we will look at the reasoning involved in the use of guidelines, scores and clinical decision aids for both clinicians and patients. We will also consider how their use can inform decision-making, leading to more reliable diagnoses, more rational investigation and more appropriate management decisions.

Many clinical guidelines, scores and decision aids function as heuristics, with the advantage of being externally constructed, usually incorporating the best evidence available and the consensus of a medical community about their validity and reliability. The intention of all of them is to increase the likelihood of patients receiving evidence-based care, with presumed benefits to patients in terms of outcomes and to healthcare systems in terms of efficiency. The benefits for healthcare professionals are increased confidence that good care is being provided, and in time saved as a result of the critical appraisal and synthesis of research evidence being done by external bodies.

## Clinical guidelines

The development of a clinical guideline begins with a systematic review of the literature on the topic being considered. The process is at risk of bias and conflicts of interest, and a well-conducted systematic review will include a description of how this risk has been addressed. It must also include assessments of the strength of the evidence from each piece of research. Subsequent steps involve consultation with a wide variety of stakeholders, including patient representatives, before the guideline is made available to clinicians. There are many guidelines available, and it can be difficult for clinicians to judge which are the best ones to use.

One of the most important aspects of a clinical guideline is that its use should be demonstrated to improve outcomes for patients in real situations by means of a prospective validation study. The other features of a good clinical guideline are shown in Box 8.1.

Key decisions that clinicians must make when using clinical guidelines are about how well the guideline 'fits' the individual patient, and how population-level data translate to individuals.

## Scores and decision aids

The development of scores and decision aids involves a lengthy process starting with the identification of predictors from clinical observation, validation of the 'rules' involving cohort studies or controlled trials, analysis of the usefulness of the rule in terms of its acceptability, feasibility and cost-benefit, and then encouraging its adoption into standard clinical practice (see 'Further reading/resources'). As is also true for clinical guidelines, this last phase can be difficult as there is often resistance from clinicians to use them, probably arising from uncertainty about how to use them, doubts about their validity and reliability, and belief in the powers of 'clinical judgement' in assessing variable presentations of illness.

There are many examples of clinical decision aids, and most clinicians will be familiar with their use. A key consideration of the role they play in decision-making is knowing in what circumstances to apply them. This, in turn, depends on an accurate *clinical assessment* through the use of good consultation skills. When used judiciously, clinical decision aids can enhance a clinical decision by adding to its reliability and its acceptability to patients.

*ABC of Clinical Reasoning*, First Edition. Edited by Nicola Cooper and John Frain.
© 2017 John Wiley & Sons, Ltd. Published 2017 by John Wiley & Sons, Ltd.

Box 8.1 **Features of a good clinical guideline**

- It is based on a well-conducted and transparent systematic review that includes statements about potential conflicts of interest and about the strength of the evidence.
- A range of relevant professionals have been involved in its development and have reached a consensus about the content and recommendations.
- Patient representatives have been involved in its development and their views on its acceptability have been incorporated.
- A positive impact on outcomes for patients is likely as a result of its use.
- The guideline is applicable to an appropriate range of clinical situations and individual patients.
- The guideline is clearly written and states precisely what its recommendations are and in what circumstances they apply.
- There is enough flexibility in the guidance that patients' views and values can be taken into account.
- The guideline is updated as new evidence emerges.
- It represents a cost-effective use of resources.

There are a number of situations in which clinical decision aids may be of use:

- To inform decisions about investigations and therapeutic interventions.
- To screen for specific conditions that need a complex or costly assessment.
- When the clinical decision is a particularly complex one.

All make use of clinical assessment findings, and some include numerical scoring systems linked to these findings.

One example of a commonly used score/decision aid in clinical practice is the Wells' score for the investigation of deep vein thrombosis (DVT), in which combining history and physical examination into a numerical score is used to estimate pre-test probability, which in turn informs the decision about whether to take blood for a D-dimer test. The combination of a low Wells' score and a negative D-dimer eliminates the need for further investigations (e.g. Doppler ultrasound) in suspected DVT.

The Ottawa Ankle Rule is a decision aid that only uses clinical examination findings (Figure 8.1). When applied to the assessment of ankle injuries, it can reduce the number of unnecessary X-rays for a very common injury, by selecting a specific population (those with a defined group of physical signs on examination) in which the prevalence of fracture is higher. This increases the positive predictive value of the test, and by the correct application of the rules, exposure to radiation and expenditure on X-rays can be reduced.

Other clinical decision aids use the presence or absence of defined symptoms as the basis for predicting the likelihood of a specific diagnosis. The Rome II criteria for irritable bowel syndrome is an example of a clinical decision aid that uses verbal descriptors and concentrates predominantly on the patient's symptoms (see Box 8.2).

The Wells' score, Ottawa Ankle Rule and the Rome II criteria all play an important part in the rational use of investigations in defined circumstances.

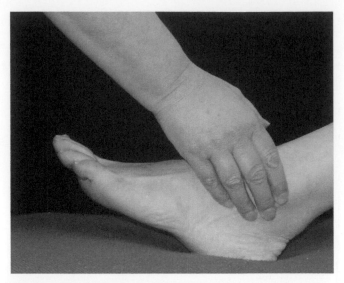

**Figure 8.1** Examination of the ankle using the Ottawa Ankle Rule. The Ottawa Ankle Rule has a high sensitivity and moderate specificity, therefore a very low rate of false negatives. The original study reported that the Rule was 100% sensitive and reduced the number of ankle X-rays by 36% – subsequent larger trials replicated these findings. (Stiell IG, Greenberg GH, McKnight RD et al. A study to develop clinical decision rules for the use of radiography in acute ankle injuries. *Ann Emerg Med* 1992; **21**:384–90.)

Box 8.2 **The Rome II criteria for diagnosing irritable bowel syndrome**

The diagnosis of a functional bowel disorder always presumes the absence of a structural or biochemical explanation for the symptoms.

At least 12 weeks, which need not be consecutive, in the preceding 12 months of abdominal discomfort or pain that has two out of three features:

- Relieved with defecation
- Onset associated with a change in frequency of stool
- Onset associated with a change in form (appearance) of stool

Symptoms that cumulatively support the diagnosis of irritable bowel syndrome:

- Abnormal stool frequency (for research purposes 'abnormal' may be defined as greater than three bowel movements per day or fewer than three bowel movements per week)
- Abnormal stool form (lumpy/hard or loose/watery stool)
- Abnormal stool passage (straining, urgency, or feeling of incomplete evacuation)
- Passage of mucus
- Bloating or feeling of abdominal distension

Reproduced with permission of the Rome Foundation.

## The pitfalls of using guidelines, scores and decision aids

Despite their advantages, there are also pitfalls in using guidelines and clinical decision aids (Box 8.3). The difficulty with guidelines is that they are based on evidence from studies of large groups of people. A key clinical decision is how applicable they are to an

Box 8.3 **The pitfalls of using clinical guidelines and decision aids**

Possible pitfalls of using clinical guidelines and decision aids are:

- Screening tools are erroneously used for diagnosis.
- Assumptions that all diseases present and progress in a uniform manner.
- Application of population-level findings to individuals.
- Failure to take patient factors and preferences into account.

Box 8.4 **Sackett et al.'s definition of evidence-based medicine**

'Evidence-based medicine is the integration of best (current) research evidence with clinical expertise and patient values.'

From Sackett DL, Rosenberg WM, Gray JA, Haynes RB, Richardson WS. Evidence-based medicine: what it is and what it isn't. *BMJ* 1996; **312**:71–2.

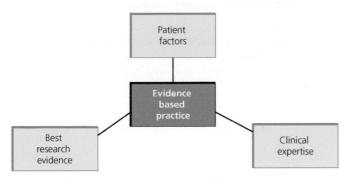

**Figure 8.2** Evidence-based practice.

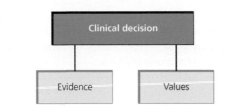

**Figure 8.3** Values-based practice and the 'two feet' principle.

Box 8.5 **An example of the inappropriate use of guidelines**

Mrs H was a 92-year-old woman who had a total hip replacement after a fall 2 months previously, with an episode of acute renal failure post-operatively from which she made a good recovery. Blood tests on discharge showed that her renal function was back to previous levels (eGFR 52 mL/min/1.73 m$^2$) and her haemoglobin level was 120 g/L. She never required a blood transfusion during her hospital stay. She presented to her general practitioner (GP) complaining of weakness.

The GP repeated her blood tests:

- Haemoglobin (Hb) 110 g/L (115–165 g/L)
- Mean corpuscular volume (MCV) 79 fL (80–96 fL)
- Mean corpuscular haemoglobin (MCH) 25 pg (28–32 pg)
- Serum iron 45 mcg/dL (50–170 mcg/dL)
- eGFR 50 mL/min/1.73 m$^2$

The GP interpreted these results as indicating iron deficiency anaemia, then considered this in the light of guidelines for the investigation of iron deficiency anaemia in an elderly woman and decided to refer her for gastroenterological assessment.

Mrs H agreed after much persuasion by her family to follow the GP's advice. She underwent a gastroscopy and colonoscopy, finding the tests unpleasant and painful. No abnormalities were found.

In the follow-up appointment, Mrs H described a low mood and a feeling of being a burden to her family and to the National Health Service. She admitted that she wanted to die. She was noted to be unkempt with uncombed hair. The GP undertook an assessment on her mental state using a standard instrument. The score suggested depression, and an appropriate antidepressant medication was started. The side effects of this medication caused her to have an episode of haematemesis requiring another hospital stay.

One month later, there was no improvement. Mrs H complained about pain in her jaw when she chewed, and this had been preventing her from eating for some months. Her arms felt too weak to lift them and combing her hair was making her scalp hurt. The GP took blood to measure her erythrocyte sedimentation rate, which was raised, and as a result diagnosed polymyalgia rheumatica with temporal arteritis. Treatment with an appropriate dose of prednisolone (with a proton pump inhibitor) resulted in a dramatic recovery of both her physical and mental symptoms.

individual patient, in terms of the specific and often unique set of circumstances for that patient from a disease perspective, and also in terms of what their personal ideas and preferences are. Sackett, the 'father of evidence-based medicine', sums this up in Box 8.4, and Figure 8.2 is a graphic representation of his definition.

Another way of looking at this is the concept of *values-based practice*. One aspect of this is that any clinical decision rests on two 'feet' – scientific evidence and the values of patients and their carers, even when the decision does not, at first glance, seem to be heavily value laden to the consulting clinician (Figure 8.3).

In applying a guideline without taking these individual factors into account, outcomes may not be optimal. Patients may be subjected to procedures and treatments that are inappropriate for them in their circumstances or unacceptable to them for a variety of reasons, even though they happen to meet 'the criteria'. Either circumstance may result in harm.

Box 8.5 describes a series of events in which guidelines were applied and a clinical scoring system used without a proper consideration of all the relevant factors relating to the patient. If a full history had been taken at the time of her first presentation, the cardinal symptoms of polymyalgia rheumatica and temporal arteritis would have emerged, and her blood tests could have been interpreted in the light of that diagnostic hypothesis, leading to an appropriate management decision. The doctor in this case used pattern recognition without pausing to analyse his assumptions and thinking, a pitfall described in previous chapters. Heuristics (pattern recognition), which might have been appropriate in a different situation, were applied erroneously, leading to a delayed diagnosis and harm to the patient. She endured unnecessary gastroenterological investigations, side effects from inappropriate medication, and a delayed diagnosis.

Sometimes, clinical decision aids are used to make a diagnosis when they were designed as screening tools. This is inappropriate and can lead to misleading results. The correct approach would dictate that a positive result should lead to a deeper clinical assessment before a diagnosis is made. An example of this is the CAGE Questionnaire (see 'Further reading/resources'), which was intended to be a screening tool for alcohol dependence, and makes use of four questions to be asked during medical history taking. A score of 2 or more is associated with problem drinking and is a cue to explore drinking habits further – it does not diagnose alcoholism. It is important that such tools are used for the purpose for which they were designed and in the context of a fuller clinical assessment.

Some decision aids take the form of algorithms and are often electronically based. While they can help with some aspects of making decisions, they rely on classical presentations and progression of disease and cannot take into account individual variation and anomalies, and thus involve the potential for errors.

## Applying clinical guidelines in practice – helping patients to share decision-making

As we have seen, clinical communication is a vital part of using guidelines in clinical practice. This communication needs to be directed at reaching a shared understanding with patients about their illness in order to share decision-making with them. Clinicians need to be able to translate scientific, population-based data into a practical management plan for the patient in front of them. This involves many complex decisions, relating (i) to the critical appraisal of the information itself and its practical application, (ii) to the assessment of the needs of the patient and (iii) how to maximise the chances of the patient accepting and adhering to the proposed management plan. The decisions involved in this latter aspect are about how to communicate risks and benefits of treatments to patients. There is evidence that many people do not understand percentages, proportions or ratios, and that a more effective strategy is to use 'absolute risk'. For example, when thinking about women deciding whether or not to take hormone replacement therapy because of the risk of breast cancer, consider the three statements in Box 8.6. They all sound quite different, and it may be difficult to know what each actually means.

Now consider the statements in Box 8.7. This is the same risk expressed as the absolute risk and is much easier to understand. Patients are likely to feel more confident about making a decision having been given the information in this form.

Another way of using absolute risk is by talking about absolute risk reduction, and a variation of this is the concept of 'prolongation of life'. This can be used when helping patients to decide about preventative measures such as stopping smoking. Consider the case in Box 8.8, for example.

As a result of the patient having information as a simple statement of prolongation of life, she was able to understand the benefits of stopping smoking in a way that was directly related to her concerns, and could perceive a clear and easily comprehensible gain if she could manage to stop. This increased her conviction that she should stop. The doctor used reasoning skills to make decisions

---

**Box 8.6 Talking about risk and hormone replacement therapy (HRT)**

- For women who take HRT, the risk of breast cancer increases by almost one-third.
- For women who take HRT, the risk of breast cancer increases by 26%.
- For women who take HRT, the risk of breast cancer is 1.26 times greater than for those who do not take HRT.

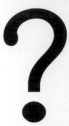

---

**Box 8.7 Talking about *absolute risk* and hormone replacement therapy (HRT)**

- In a group of 1000 women, there will be three new cases of breast cancer every year.
- In a group of 1000 women who take HRT, there will be nearly four new cases of breast cancer every year.

---

**Box 8.8 Using 'prolongation of life' to encourage smoking cessation**

- Donna is 40 years old. She has smoked 25 cigarettes a day since she was 16. Donna's general practitioner (GP) wants to convey to her the benefits of stopping smoking.
- The GP knows that the chance of a woman who smokes surviving until the age of 79 years is 32% lower than for one who does not, and that the rate of death from any cause amongst current smokers is three times higher for people aged 25 to 79 years than for those who do not smoke. The GP also knows that the average age of death for women who do not smoke is 81 years, and 71 years for those who do smoke. The absolute risk reduction (for dying from a cause associated with smoking) is 90% for those who stop smoking before they are 40 years old. Donna has not been convinced by any of these arguments. She thinks that she has smoked for so long that nothing will make any difference now.
- The GP decides to try a different approach. She wants to convey to Donna that stopping smoking will have a positive effect on her life expectancy. After some searching, she finds out that if Donna were to stop smoking in the next year, she is likely to live for about nine years longer than if she does not stop. This would mean that her life expectancy would become almost the same as if she had never smoked.
- Donna found this information compelling, worked hard at stopping smoking and was successful. She also convinced her partner to stop by using the same argument.

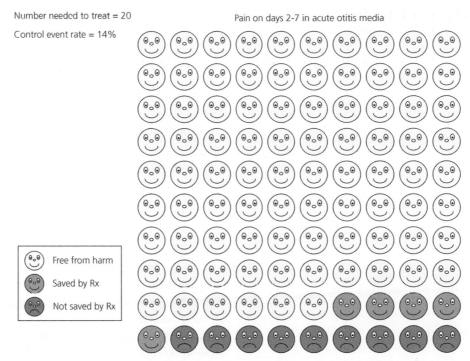

Number needed to treat = 20

Control event rate = 14%

Pain on days 2-7 in acute otitis media

Free from harm

Saved by Rx

Not saved by Rx

**Figure 8.4** Portrayal of risks and benefits of treatment with antibiotics for otitis media designed with 'Visual Rx', a program that calculates numbers needed to treat from the pooled results of a meta-analysis and produces a graphical display of the result. From Edwards A, Elwyn G and Mulley A. Explaining risks: turning numerical data into meaningful pictures. *BMJ* 2002; **324**:827–30. Reproduced with permission from BMJ Publishing Group Ltd.

about how to find, appraise, interpret and apply evidence-based information to achieve a good outcome for the patient.

In recent years, extending the concept of giving patients enough information to make informed decisions about their health has led to a growing interest in formal Patient Decision Aids (PDAs). These are intended to present evidence-based information to patients in a way they can easily understand in order to help them make decisions with the support of their clinician. An example of such a decision aid is shown in Figure 8.4. This is intended to help a clinician reach a shared decision with a patient about the treatment of acute otitis media with antibiotics. The information is simple and visual and helps both patient and clinician to make a management decision.

There is currently rapid development in the field of patient decision aids that goes hand in hand with the democratisation of data as a result of better access via electronic means. Patients will often arrive in their consultations with ideas generated as a result of their own searches. An important contributor to many consultations is the clinician's willingness to help with the interpretation of such information and its application to the patient's individual circumstances.

## Summary

Clinical decision-making can be supported by using a variety of guidelines, scoring systems and descriptive criteria-based tools. These can help with diagnostic and management decisions, both

regarding the rationality of testing and therapeutic planning. These decision aids must be applied and interpreted *within the context of a comprehensive clinical assessment*, which requires good history taking, examination and communication skills.

Once the diagnosis is made, clinical decision-making continues and becomes the shared responsibility of the clinician and the patient. There are specific decision-making skills involved in this part of the consultation, in which scientific knowledge must be combined with the patient's values and wishes.

## Further reading/resources

Adams ST and Leveson SH. Clinical prediction rules. *BMJ* 2012; **344**:d8312.

Ewing J. Detecting alcoholism: the CAGE questionnaire. *JAMA* 1984; **252**:1905–7.

National Institute for Health and Care Excellence. Venous thromboembolic diseases: the management of venous thromboembolic diseases and the role of thrombophilia testing. NICE clinical guideline number 144, 2012. Available at: www.nice.org.uk/guidance/cg144 (accessed 23 February 2016).

Peile E. Teaching balanced clinical decision-making in primary care: evidence-based and values based approaches used in conjunction. *Educ Prim Care* 2014; **25**:67–70.

Sackett DL, Rosenberg WM, Gray JA, Haynes RB, Richardson WS. Evidence-based medicine: what it is and what it isn't. *BMJ* 1996; **312**(7023):71–2.

Shekelle PG, Woolf SH, Eccles M, Grimshaw J. Developing guidelines. *BMJ* 1999; **318**:593–6. [Part of a four article series on the development and use of clinical guidelines.]

# CHAPTER 9

# Teaching Clinical Reasoning

*Nicola Cooper[1], Ana L. Da Silva[2] and Sian Powell[3]*

[1] Derby Teaching Hospitals NHS Foundation Trust; and University of Nottingham, UK
[2] Swansea University Medical School, Swansea, UK
[3] Imperial College School of Medicine, Charing Cross Hospital, London, UK

---

## OVERVIEW

- Sound clinical reasoning is directly linked to patient safety and quality of care
- A shared vocabulary and understanding of key concepts is a starting point for teaching and learning clinical reasoning
- Evidence from cognitive psychology, education and studies of expertise give us an insight into how learning clinical reasoning can be facilitated
- There is no evidence that short courses improve clinical reasoning skills – teaching and learning should be integrated throughout an entire curriculum
- The most effective way to gain clinical reasoning skills is by practice on actual or hypothetical cases, combined with feedback and reflection

## Introduction

As outlined in Chapter 1, diagnostic error is common and causes significant harm. In a study of diagnostic error in internal medicine, the most common root causes of diagnostic error were system-related factors and human cognitive error – either the data were not gathered optimally or the available data were not synthesised correctly. Undergraduate and postgraduate training programmes now teach the science behind patient safety and human factors, addressing system-related and communication factors that lead to error. But less attention has been paid to clinical reasoning and decision-making.

Clinical reasoning should not be seen as an 'add on' to any curriculum, requiring more teaching time. Instead, we need to consider how what is already in place can be realigned to facilitate teaching and learning in this important area. The authors Rencic, Trowbridge and Durning (see 'Further reading/ resources') say that clinical reasoning's broad and fundamental nature means 'it is housed nowhere but should be taught everywhere' and should be treated as a foundational science

like anatomy and physiology, explicitly integrated into various courses throughout undergraduate and postgraduate training.

However, there are challenges; in particular the challenge of equipping every clinical teacher with the knowledge and skills required to teach clinical reasoning. This can be overcome in part by using a core group of experienced clinician-educators to teach key parts of the curriculum and to provide training in simple techniques for other clinical teachers. This chapter outlines some recommendations for teaching clinical reasoning based on available evidence, studies of expertise, and educational theories relevant to clinical reasoning.

## A spiral curriculum

The term 'spiral curriculum' refers to a process whereby topics are revisited over time with increasing levels of difficulty, with new information, new applications and further practical experience.

A starting point for teaching and learning clinical reasoning is a shared vocabulary among teachers and learners and an understanding of key concepts. While a vast knowledge of medicine is required for excellent clinical reasoning, there are key concepts specific to clinical reasoning that can form a syllabus (an outline of the subjects to be taught) for learning in this area. This is shown in Table 9.1.

In the first two to three years of undergraduate studies, teaching should focus on straightforward presentations of common diseases. Learning prototypal presentations of common diseases helps learners build a database of 'illness scripts' that can be added to with increasing complexity throughout their training, and is an important foundation for the development of their pattern recognition abilities. This can be done through case discussions as well as real patients. Key teaching points for each presentation should be established to ensure consistency. Students should be encouraged to synthesise data they gather from history, examination and initial test results into a *problem list* (e.g. 'weight loss and microcytic anaemia') rather than moving straight to a differential

---

**Table 9.1** Key topics in a clinical reasoning syllabus.

| Topic | Sub-topic |
|---|---|
| Clinical skills | Effective communication |
| | Evidence-based history |
| | Evidence-based examination |
| | Shared decision-making |
| | Communicating risk |
| Probability | Odds ratios |
| | Likelihood ratios |
| | Pre-test and post-test probability |
| | Principles of Bayes' theorem |
| Using and interpreting diagnostic tests | Clinical probability |
| | Sensitivity and specificity |
| | Predictive values |
| | Factors other than disease that influence test results |
| | Commonly used tests (by specialty) to illustrate important principles. For example, in internal medicine: |
| | • D-dimer |
| | • Urinalysis in suspected urinary tract infections |
| | • 12-lead electrocardiogram in chest pain |
| | • Spirometry in suspected COPD |
| | • Ultrasound in abdominal pain |
| | • Computed tomography in suspected stroke |
| Models of clinical reasoning | The difference between deductive and inductive reasoning |
| | Abductive reasoning |
| | Probabilistic reasoning |
| | Causal reasoning |
| | Dual process theory/universal model of diagnostic reasoning (see Chapter 4) |
| Cognitive biases and errors | Definitions |
| | Common cognitive biases |
| Human factors | The limitations of human performance |
| | Affective biases |
| | Effective communication in teams |
| | SBAR (see Chapter 6) |
| Metacognition and cognitive debiasing | Understanding when type 1 and type 2 thinking is being used |
| | Traditional debiasing methods (see Chapter 7) |
| | Checklists |
| | Evidence-based medicine |
| | Use of guidelines, scores and decision aids |
| | Pitfalls of using guidelines, scores and decision aids inappropriately |
| Learning clinical reasoning | Deliberate practice theory |
| | How we organise and store knowledge effectively |
| | Reflection |

diagnosis (e.g. 'it could be stomach cancer') as this can be used to teach important clinical reasoning steps, such as:

• Identification of key clinical data.
• Semantic competence (the use of precise medical language important in 'chunking' information into larger units, which helps to organise and store information).
• Synthesising data into problems (or 'problem representation' – a short summary defining the case).
• Making relevant associations between problems.

• Critical thinking – for example, spotting and avoiding assumptions.
• Formulation of a management plan that takes all the patient's problems into account.

At this stage, basic clinical reasoning concepts can be introduced, such as evidence-based history and examination, use and interpretation of diagnostic tests, probabilistic reasoning, common cognitive biases, using guidelines, scores and decision aids, and shared decision-making with patients. While lectures on the important concepts of clinical reasoning play a role, this is not the most effective way to learn. Small group case-based discussions and discussing a patient the student has just seen is likely to be more effective. Again, key teaching points should be established to ensure consistency.

In the final years of undergraduate studies and in early postgraduate training, learners have substantially more clinical experience, and teaching should shift to consolidating their knowledge and giving as much opportunity as possible to reflect on their own clinical reasoning through seeing as many patients as possible and participating in individual or group case-based discussions. Emphasis should be placed on building knowledge of atypical presentations of common diseases and typical presentations of uncommon diseases. For this to be effective, a breadth of clinical experience is required and clinical attachments should emphasise the clinical reasoning process.

At this stage, students can be taught about dual process theory and specific strategies to use when in each mode of thinking; they can practise their pattern recognising skills while understanding the effect of cognitive biases on their decision-making; they can learn about debiasing strategies and receive training in human factors. From this point on, new information is continually being added to an expanding database of 'illness scripts' and clinical reasoning skills are being refined.

An illustration of a spiral curriculum in clinical reasoning is shown in Figure 9.1.

## Educational theories relevant to clinical reasoning

### How knowledge is organised

Clinical reasoning is not a stand-alone skill – it is highly dependent on knowledge and knowledge organisation. Therefore students should be encouraged in methods that help them amass as much organised knowledge as possible. The human brain has limited short-term memory. To overcome this limitation, clinicians 'chunk' information into larger units. The use of precise medical terms, problem representations and illness scripts are examples of how experts chunk knowledge (see Table 9.2). Chunking uses long-term working memory, which is believed to have endless capacity. Experienced clinicians use chunking to process and retrieve information efficiently. Learners can be encouraged to use chunking, as the example in Box 9.1 illustrates.

Illness scripts are the product of extensive experience with patients combined with formal knowledge. The clinical reasoning of students is characterised by poorly organised knowledge. Expert clinicians, on the other hand, use illness scripts most of the time in

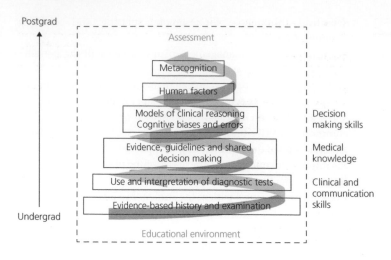

**Figure 9.1** A spiral curriculum for clinical reasoning. In a spiral curriculum, topics are continually revisited with increasing levels of difficulty throughout one's training and clinical practice.

**Table 9.2** 'Chunking' information into larger units – for example, precise medical terms, problem representation and illness scripts. A 'chunk' can vary in complexity from a semantic qualifier to a complex illness script.

| Term | Definition |
|---|---|
| Precise medical terms (also known as 'semantic qualifiers') | A binary, abstract descriptor – for example, acute or chronic, colicky or constant, pleuritic or dull |
| Summary statements (problem representation) | A single sentence that incorporates clinical context, temporal pattern and pertinent clinical findings – for example, a 60-year-old man with new onset cardiac-sounding chest pain on minimal exertion |
| Illness scripts | A medical schema (representation or conceptual framework) – for example, strep throat = exudative pharyngitis, fever, lymphadenopathy, and lack of cough |

Adapted from Ratcliffe TA and Durning SJ. Theoretical concepts to consider in providing clinical reasoning instruction. In: Trowbridge RI, Rencic JJ and Durning SJ. *Teaching Clinical Reasoning*. Philadelphia: American College of Physicians, 2015.

their clinical reasoning and use a knowledge-driven model of forward thinking and pattern recognition that is more efficient than the hypothesis testing used most by students (see Figures 9.2 and 9.3). As learners acquire more clinical experience, they can be coached in using the strategies that experts use.

Illness scripts are continually refined throughout one's medical training. Building illness scripts can be encouraged by:
- Seeing as many patients/discussing as many cases as possible.
- Effective chunking.
- Reading strategically.

When learners read about their patients' problems in context (e.g. after seeing the patient that day), this promotes conceptualisation rather than memorisation, and textbook knowledge is organised in a way that is more likely to be recalled.

Another way to facilitate the organisation of knowledge is through the use of concept maps (or trees), which can help learners encapsulate and organise knowledge in a way that is clinically relevant. Concept maps are different from mind maps.

**Box 9.1 Encouraging semantic competence/accurate problem representation**

One of the authors was teaching a final year medical student who had just 'clerked in' an elderly woman with acute confusion. The student had followed his brief and had phoned the patient's husband for an eyewitness account of what had been happening at home. After getting the history, examining the patient and reviewing the initial test results, the student created a problem list:

Problem 1: acute confusion
Problem 2: raised creatinine

The student's plan for each problem was extremely woolly. But when the student was encouraged to describe the patient's problems using more precise medical terms he was able to redefine them as:

Problem 1: delirium
Problem 2: acute kidney injury

After defining the problems using more precise medical terms, the student was quickly able to retrieve relevant information from previous learning and create a comprehensive management plan for each problem. The student was encouraged to read up on delirium after seeing this particular patient to consolidate his knowledge.

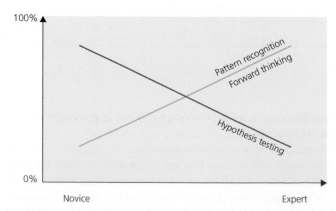

**Figure 9.2** Expert clinicians mainly use forward thinking and pattern recognition, which is more efficient than the hypothesis testing used by novices.

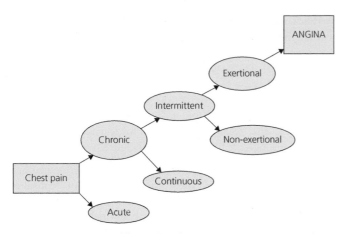

**Figure 9.3** An example of forward thinking.

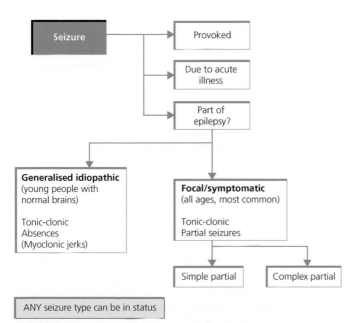

**Figure 9.4** An example of a concept map (or tree) used in teaching, to facilitate organised learning and memory in what can appear to be a complex clinical topic.

They are a way to develop logical thinking and learning by illustrating connections and helping students see how individual problems form part of a larger whole. They are constructed to reflect organisation of memory, and therefore facilitate learners' ability to make sense of things, which aids meaningful learning. An example of how this can be used in teaching is given in Figure 9.4.

### Deliberate practice and the development of expertise

We know from studies of expertise that key ingredients in the development of expert professional practice are experience (lots of it), coupled with deliberate practice, coaching and feedback, and the ability to reflect and learn from mistakes. Therefore, facilitating coaching and feedback is extremely important but can also be challenging. Deliberate practice theory suggests that more learning would take place by working with a limited number of

**Table 9.3** Applying theory to teach clinical reasoning.

| Teaching tip | Theoretical basis |
|---|---|
| Be explicit about building knowledge and knowledge organisation<br>• Store and retrieve facts about diseases as illness scripts<br>• Connect and apply stored knowledge including biomedical knowledge | Information processing |
| Identify and accurately represent problems<br>• Use semantic qualifiers<br>• Develop summary statements | |
| Develop both non-analytical and analytical reasoning skills<br>Think fast:<br>• Pattern recognition<br>• Intuition and heuristics<br>Think slow:<br>• Hypothetico-deduction<br>• Probabilistic (Bayesian) reasoning | |
| Foster motivation to monitor and improve reasoning<br>• Commit to most likely diagnosis<br>• Try to predict diagnostic test results | Deliberate practice<br>Self-regulated learning |
| Seek and provide timely feedback on reasoning<br>• Use test results or clinical course as source of feedback<br>• Analyse and reflect on successes and failures in clinical reasoning | |
| Create opportunities for further practice and incremental improvement<br>• Apply reasoning to new patients or problems<br>• Practice harder: increase complexity; manage uncertainty/ambiguity; reason despite incomplete data | |

Reproduced with permission from Ledford CH and Nixon LJ. General teaching techniques. In: Trowbridge RL, Rencic JJ and Durning SJ (eds), *Teaching Clinical Reasoning*. Philadelphia: American College of Physicians, 2015.

experienced coaches for a period than by working with a different clinician every day or clinical attachments that change every few weeks.

A summary of how to apply theory to teaching clinical reasoning is shown in Table 9.3.

### Teaching techniques

Educational activities need to start by developing a common language and shared understanding of key concepts in clinical reasoning. These will probably take place in a tutorial-type format as the goal is primarily to share knowledge. However, learning clinical reasoning requires ongoing practical engagement.

Short courses designed to train novices in decision-making and cognitive biases are ineffective. As the authors Del Mar, Doust and Glasziou (see 'Further reading/resources') state:

> There is evidence that the most effective way for students to gain diagnostic skills is by practice on actual or hypothetical cases, while receiving feedback on their performance. Essential features appear to be both the practical experience

(the gaining of stories and prototypes) and the feedback (so that abstract models and generalisations can be acquired). Students need to be exposed to a wide variety of common presentations and spectra of disease, so that they can acquire the 'illness scripts' necessary to be able to come to a diagnosis. Using simulated cases with the explicit explanation of hypothesis testing and refinement and gradual release of findings, allowing students to practice their clinical reasoning appears effective. Students [also] need to gain feedback in a wide variety of clinical contexts … as there is evidence that it is difficult to transfer clinical reasoning from one context to another.

The following techniques have been described in the literature.

## Case-based interventions

*Problem-solving clinical seminars* – groups of learners are expected to analyse one or more clinical cases in advance and discuss questions with a focus on clinical reasoning skills.

*Diagnostic grand rounds* – these are sessions in which experts introduce clinical cases, sharing reasoning strategies as more clinical information is revealed. In one study, almost 400 final-year students covered 23 clinical cases using this format. The effect on their clinical reasoning was measured by a before-and-after score on the Diagnostic Thinking Inventory (DTI), a self-reported measure of individual clinical reasoning characteristics. The results showed an increase in clinical reasoning flexibility and structure (Stieger S, Praschinger A, Kletter K et al. Diagnostic grand rounds: a new teaching concept to train diagnostic reasoning. *Eur J Radiol* 2011; 78(3):349–52).

*Integrated case learning* – this activity starts with a clinical encounter that is role played by a clinician-educator while students observe. Two students share the role of 'doctor' in the situation while others take on different clinical reasoning roles. As the case progresses, uncertainties are revealed and discussed, a differential diagnosis is generated, investigations are analysed and possible pathways are justified by the 'doctors' to the rest of the group. Qualitative analysis of these activities shows this process appears to stimulate clinical reasoning and contributes towards the transition to clinical practice.

*Simulation and debriefings* – these activities use high-fidelity simulation scenarios followed by a debriefing in which learners are given the opportunity to discuss their performance. In emergency medicine, this has been used to develop clinical reasoning skills. Simulation is already widespread in teaching emergency drills and human factors.

*Virtual learning patients* – this refers to computer programs that simulate real-life clinical scenarios. Analysis of this technique shows it has a positive effect on the development of clinical reasoning skills, but no difference when compared with other non-computer interventions. Interventions that rely on information technology can be resource intensive but there are now several providers to which medical schools can subscribe – http://openlabyrinth.ca and www.med-u.org/fmcases are examples (accessed February 2016).

## Reflection and metacognition strategies

Learners require lots of clinical experience because clinical reasoning ability is influenced by the case and the context in which it occurs. The more diverse cases that learners are exposed to, the better they are prepared to solve new cases. Reflection, self-assessment and the ability to identify one's own learning needs are associated with the development of expertise in medicine, so interventions that create opportunities for learners to engage in effective reflection are likely to improve clinical reasoning skills.

*Time outs* – these are used in role plays, simulation or planned clinical encounters in which the learner is observed in a consultation and stopped at key moments. The situation is 'frozen' while the facilitator or group asks the learner about their decisions and actions – 'Why did you ask that question?', 'What hypothesis are you testing there?'

*One Minute Preceptor* – this is a work-based teaching technique, used when a learner has just seen a patient. It consists of five steps that encourage the learner to 'own' the problem and identify gaps in their knowledge:
- Get the learner to commit to what they think is going on.
- Probe for supporting evidence, why they made that decision.
- Teach one or two general principles.
- Reinforce what was done well.
- Correct one or two errors in reasoning.

*Cognitive forcing strategies* – (see Chapter 7) these are strategies to allow clinicians to self-monitor their own thinking, and can be used in teaching as well.

## Reflection in clinical reasoning

Compelling theoretical evidence exists to suggest that clinicians reflect to solve difficult problems in practice, and that this is one way in which their expertise develops. Donald Schön was particularly influential in describing what experts do when they are faced with 'a disorientating dilemma' in which they are unable to rely on tacit knowledge or non-analytical reasoning strategies to solve the problem as they would in routine practice. Instead, according to Schön, experts engage first in 'reflection-in-action' to make sense of the encounter, and later 'reflection-on-action' to learn from the encounter and enhance their clinical expertise.

Schön's main contribution was the idea that reflection (see Box 9.2) could have an immediate significance for action. Most reflective learning tools used for teaching and learning facilitate retrospective reflection, for example case-based discussions and significant event analyses. However, Schön suggested that reflection *during* a clinical encounter can change and improve the outcome of the encounter as it is occurring in real time. Clinicians

---

Box 9.2 **Reflection-in-action 1**

'Reflection is a metacognitive process that occurs before, during or after situations with the purpose of developing greater understanding of both self and the situation to inform future actions.'

Sandars J. The use of reflection in medical education. AMEE Guide no. 44. *Medical Teacher* 2009; **31**:685–95.

who are 'reflecting-in-action' are more likely to notice when something is out of the ordinary and can then choose to pause to think about their thinking – whether their current reasoning strategy is adequate, and whether their thinking is influenced by bias (see Box 9.3).

As a consequence, it has been suggested that reflection can be thought of as a learning strategy that can be used during uncertain and complex clinical encounters. The 'Stop and Think' framework (see Figure 9.5) is a reflective learning tool that can guide and facilitate 'reflection-in-action' during clinical encounters. It is designed to prompt the activities described by Schön, and also framed within a hypothetico-deductive model taught in medical schools. The framework can be used whenever a clinician

### Box 9.3 **Reflection-in-action 2**

Reflection during clinical case-solving can help clinicians to:

- Notice when something is out of the ordinary, 'stop and think' and switch from non-analytical to analytical reasoning
- Think about their thinking – Am I being comprehensive? Have I missed something? Is my judgement affected by bias?
- Make thought processes explicit. This facilitates creation of shared management plans with patients and enables critical appraisal
- Cope with complexity – by utilising analytical thought processes and taking time to make sense of a difficult situation
- Cope with uncertainty – by considering worse case scenarios and ensuring a safety net and plan for monitoring
- Learn from difficult situations and increase clinical expertise

---

**'Stop and think' framework**

**Name the problem**

- What have I noticed?
- What are my initial thoughts?
- What are my underlying feelings about the situation?

**Reframe the problem**

- How else can I think of this problem?
- What have I already identified?
- What is the likely effect of this problem?

**Generate hypotheses**

- What else could be going on? (Consider surgical sieve, pathophysiological mechanisms, epidemiology, patient co-morbidities and medications, psychological factors, context)
- What is the worse case scenario?

**Deduct hypotheses**

| Hypotheses | Supportive findings? | Opposing findings? | What symptoms or signs should be present but aren't? |
|---|---|---|---|
| 1. 2. 3. | | | |

**Test working hypotheses**

- How can I verify my working hypotheses? (Further questions/examination? Investigations? Test of time? Test of treatment?)
- Is there anything I still can't explain?
- Have I considered what the patient thinks?
- Do I need to make the diagnosis now?

**Monitor and detect likely consequences**

- If my diagnosis is wrong, what are the consequences?
- How will I monitor my plan and detect any consequences?
- Have I safety-netted adequately?

**Reflection-on-action**

- Is what happened to the patient what I expected?
- What additional knowledge, information or skills do I need if I encounter a similar situation in the future?
- What have I learnt about my clinical reasoning / myself?

*Am I being affected by any bias ?*

**Figure 9.5** The 'Stop and Think' framework. Reproduced with permission of Dr S Powell from Powell SE. Feasibility study of a tool that aims to motivate medical students to reflect in their clinical practice. MA thesis, Institute of Education, 2014.

encounters a difficult clinical scenario that cannot be easily solved with non-analytic reasoning strategies such as pattern recognition, but it can also be used in group tutorials or in role plays with time outs, as described above.

## Summary

There are definitely challenges to teaching clinical reasoning, but it is possible to realign existing teaching to incorporate structure, content and techniques that emphasise clinical reasoning at the same time as imparting knowledge and clinical skills. Teaching and learning clinical reasoning has to be incorporated throughout an entire curriculum to be effective. A core group of experienced clinician-educators may be required to deliver key parts of the clinical reasoning curriculum and to provide training in simple techniques for other clinical teachers. Such training could have the advantage of helping clinicians develop their own clinical reasoning skills. The idea of a spiral curriculum is important in clinical reasoning, and there are several strategies that can be used within that to facilitate learning in this vital area of clinical practice.

## Further reading/resources

Bowen JL. Education strategies to promote clinical diagnostic reasoning. *NEJM* 2006; **355**:2217–35.

Del Mar C, Doust J, Glasziou P. *Clinical Thinking. Evidence, Communication and Decision Making.* London: Blackwell/BMJ Books, 2006.

Neher JO and Stevens N. The one minute preceptor: shaping the teaching conversation. *Fam Med* 2003; **35**(6):391–3.

Rencic J, Trowbridge RL, Durning SJ. Developing a curriculum in clinical reasoning. In: Trowbridge RL, Rencic JJ and Durning SJ (eds), *Teaching Clinical Reasoning.* Philadelphia: American College of Physicians, 2015, pp. 31–50.

Schmidt HG and Rikers RM. How expertise develops in medicine: knowledge encapsulation and illness script formation. *Med Educ* 2007; **41**:1133–9.

Schon, D. *The Reflective Practitioner: How Professionals Think in Action.* Basic Books, 1983.

Two Best Evidence Medical Education (BEME) systematic reviews are underway at the time of writing: one on 'educational interventions to promote/teach clinical reasoning' and the other on 'assessing clinical reasoning'. These will be published in 2016 on the BEME website (http://bemecollaboration.org/).

# Recommended Books, Articles and Websites

## Popular

Dobelli R. *The Art of Thinking Clearly: Better Thinking, Better Decisions*. Sceptre, 2014.

Gawande A. *The Checklist Manifesto: How to Get Things Right*. Profile Books, 2011.

Groopman J. *How Doctors Think*. Mariner Books, 2008.

Hallinan JT. *Why We Make Mistakes*. Broadway Books, 2009.

Kahneman D. *Thinking, Fast and Slow*. Penguin, 2011.

Sanders L. *Diagnosis. Dispatches From the Frontlines of Medical Mysteries*. Icon Books, 2010. [By the physician who inspired the TV show 'House'.]

Syed M. *Bounce: The Myth of Talent and the Power of Practice*. Fourth Estate, 2010.

## For students and teachers

Brush J. *The Science of the Art of Medicine*. Dementi Milestone Publishing, 2015.

Del Mar C, Doust J, Glasziou P. *Clinical thinking* BMJ-Blackwell, 2006.

Kassirer JP, Wong JB, Kopelman RI. *Learning Clinical Reasoning*, 2nd edn. Lippincott, Williams & Wilkins, 2009.

Llewelyn H, Aun Aung H, Lewis K, Al-Abdullah A. *Oxford Handbook of Clinical Diagnosis*. Oxford University Press, 2013.

McGee S. *Evidence-based Physical Diagnosis*. Saunders, 2012.

Shiralkar U. *Smart Surgeons, Sharp Decisions. Cognitive Skills to Avoid Errors and Achieve Results*. Gutenberg Press Ltd, 2011.

Sox HC, Higgins MC, Owens DK. *Medical Decision Making*, 2nd edn. Wiley-Blackwell, 2013.

Stone JV. *Bayes' Rule. A tutorial introduction to Bayesian analysis*. Sebtel Press, 2013.

Strauss SE, Richardson WS, Glasziou P, Haynes RB. *Evidence-based Medicine. How to Practice and Teach It*, 4th edn. Churchill-Livingstone, 2010.

## Academic

Hardman D. *Judgment and Decision Making: Psychological Perspectives*. Wiley, 2009.

Higgs J, Jones MA, Loftus S, Christensen N. (eds) *Clinical Reasoning in the Health Professions* 3rd edn. Elsevier, 2008.

Holyoak KJ and Morrison RG. (eds) *The Oxford Handbook of Thinking and Reasoning*. Oxford University Press, 2012.

Hunink MGM, Weinstein MC, Wittenberg E et al. *Decision Making in Health and Medicine*, 2nd edn. Cambridge University Press, 2014.

Montgomery K. *How Doctors Think. Clinical Judgement and the Practice of Medicine*. Oxford University Press, 2006.

Trowbridge RL, Rencic JJ, Durning SJ. *Teaching Clinical Reasoning*. American College of Physicians, 2015.

## Articles

Croskerry P. The importance of cognitive errors in diagnosis and strategies to minimise them. *Acad Med* 2003; **78**(8):775–80.

Croskerry P. A universal model of diagnostic reasoning. *Acad Med* 2009; **84**(8):1022–8.

Croskerry P. Bias: a normal operating characteristic of the diagnosing brain. *Diagnosis* 2014; **1**(1):23–7.

Croskerry P and Nimmo GR. Better clinical decision making and reducing diagnostic error. *J R Coll Physicians Edinb* 2011; **41**(2):155–62.

Croskerry P, Singhal G, Mamede S. Cognitive debiasing 1: origins of bias and theories of debiasing. *BMJ Qual Saf* 2013; **22**(S2):ii58–ii64.

*ABC of Clinical Reasoning*, First Edition. Edited by Nicola Cooper and John Frain.
© 2017 John Wiley & Sons, Ltd. Published 2017 by John Wiley & Sons, Ltd.

Croskerry P, Singhal G, Mamede S. Cognitive debiasing 2: impediments to and strategies for change. *BMJ Qual Saf* 2013; **22**(S2):ii65–ii72.

Dhaliwal G. The mechanics of reasoning. *JAMA* 2011; **306**(9):918–19.

Graber ML. Educational strategies to reduce diagnostic error: can you teach this stuff? *Adv Health Sci Educ* 2009; **14**:63–9.

Graber ML. Incidence of diagnostic error in medicine. *BMJ Qual Saf* 2013; **22**:ii21–ii27.

Monteiro SM and Norman G. Diagnostic reasoning: where we've been, where we're going. *Teaching and Learning in Medicine* 2013; **25**(S1):S26–32.

Norman G. The bias in researching cognitive bias. *Adv Health Sci Educ* 2014; **19**:291–5.

Scott IA. Errors in clinical reasoning: causes and remedial strategies. *BMJ* 2009; **338**:b1860.

Sherbino J and Norman GR. Reframing diagnostic error. Maybe it's content and not process that leads to error. *Acad Emerg Med* 2014; **21**(8):931–3.

Smith BW and Slack MB. The effect of cognitive debiasing training among family medicine residents. *Diagnosis* 2015; **2**(2):117–21.

## Websites (all accessed February 2016)

Institute of Medicine's 2015 report, 'Improving Diagnosis in Healthcare'
http://iom.nationalacademies.org/Reports/2015/Improving-Diagnosis-in-Healthcare/Improving-Diagnosis.aspx

Society to Improve Diagnosis in Medicine
http://www.improvediagnosis.org/

Diagnosis – an open access journal
http://www.degruyter.com/view/j/dx

IMReasoning – conversations to inspire critical thinking in clinical medicine and education
http://imreasoning.com/

Clinical Human Factors Group
http://chfg.org/

Clinical Reasoning – teaching resources
www.clinical-reasoning.org

# Index

Note: Page references in *italics* refer to Figures; those in **bold** refer to Tables and Boxes

*ABC of Clinical Reasoning*, First Edition. Edited by Nicola Cooper and John Frain.

© 2017 John Wiley & Sons, Ltd. Published 2017 by John Wiley & Sons, Ltd.

Printed and bound by CPI Group (UK) Ltd, Croydon, CR0 4YY